depression

exercise plans to improve your life

debbie lawrence and jenny burns

Other books in the *Exercise Your Way to Health* series:

Back Pain
Arthritis
Type 2 Diabetes
Osteoporosis
Stress

depression

exercise plans to improve your life

debbie lawrence and jenny burns

A & C Black • London

Published in 2011 by A&C Black Publishers Ltd
36 Soho Square, London W1D 3QY
www.acblack.com

ISBN 978 1 4081 3182 4

A CIP catalogue record for this book is available from the British Library.

Acknowledgements

Cover photograph © Shutterstock
Exercise photographs © Tom Croft
Inside photographs © Shutterstock except for those on pages
xii, 6, 14, 20, 29, 45, 56 and 99 © Getty images
Illustrations by Tom Croft, except for page 38 © Shutterstock
Designed by James Watson
Commissioned by Charlotte Croft

This book is produced using paper that is made from wood grown in managed, sustainable forests. It is natural, renewable and recyclable. The logging and manufacturing processes conform to the environmental regulations of the country of origin.

Typeset in 8.25pt Trade Gothic on 12pt by Saxon Graphics Ltd, Derby

Printed and bound in China by RR Donnelley South China Printing Co

Contents

Depression – what Winston Churchill referred to as his 'black dog'.

If your black dog is with you, remember he/she:

- needs love and TLC (not loathing)
- needs listening to even when growling (not being talked at)
- needs stroking (not bullying)
- needs coaxing in to do things (not shutting out or pushing away)
- needs small steps (rather than big leaps)
- needs encouragement and praise (not berating)
- needs empathy and warmth (not judgement and coldness)
- needs acceptance (not misunderstanding)
- needs to be experienced (not denied)

Acknowledgements

I give thanks to:

- My partner, Joe, for being the 'ray of sunshine' that he is
- Life – for the challenges it brings, which offer me the potential to continue to learn and grow
- Good health
- My mum and dad for being 'good enough' parents
- Charlotte Croft for asking me to contribute to the *Exercise Your Way to Health* series
- My co-writer, Jenny, for sharing her experience of working with people with depression to co-create this book

Debbie Lawrence

Thanks**…**

- For my husband, Rob, whose love for me has made me who I am today
- For my three beautiful sons, Robbie, Ben and Sam, who give joy beyond measure (and are growing up way too fast!)
- For the privilege of being able to help people heal on a daily basis
- To Debbie for giving me the opportunity to put into writing ways to help readers move out of depression
- To God, who underpins everything I am

Jenny Burns

The publishers would like to thank the David Lloyd Gym in Cardiff and Debbie Lawrence, Mary Sheppard, Jenny Burns, Rob Burns, Ben Burns, Mary Sparks and Paul Conway for their kind assistance with the photo-shoot.

Foreword

The benefits of exercise for our mental and physical health have been well known since ancient times. In spite of this, our society is plagued by alarming levels of illness that could have been prevented through a simple combination of good diet and exercise.

I have witnessed this development first-hand over the past 30 years as a GP in a large urban practice. Nearly 40% of our consultations are now partly or completely due to stress-related illness, anxiety and depression. I watch in dismay as our prescribing rates rise year after year in an attempt to stem this tide. But like many other doctors, I am convinced that the real cure lies in a fundamental shift away from high-tech medicine and back to basic, healthy lifestyle choices.

Many recent studies have shown exercise to be as effective as medication at beating depression. And exercise has none of the potential side effects – in fact, taking exercise also results in improved physical fitness as well as increased self-confidence and mental health. For this reason I thoroughly endorse this book. It shows in a clear and practical manner how to combat depression and anxiety with lifestyle choices and a structured exercise regime. Above all, it gives readers the tools they need to help themselves to health.

Dr P. J. Harney MB MCH MRCGP

introduction

The chances are that if you have picked up this book you want to know more for yourself about why you are feeling down or depressed. You may also be concerned about your health because you are dependant upon habits such as alcohol, drugs or cigarettes to help you cope.

This book is full of valuable information about depression and provides lots of simple and effective lifestyle tips to help improve your health and wellbeing. Most importantly, there's a section on easy exercises to do at home or at work – or wherever you happen to be. For many people, activity plays a key part in combating depression. So well done, you are taking an important first step to help manage your low moods.

It should be understood that this book is not intended to replace medical support or help. Don't be afraid to visit the doctor and discuss the way you are feeling with them. Your GP will be able to help you, providing an informed diagnosis and perhaps by prescribing anti-depressants or a talking treatment.

In the meantime getting more active and introducing exercise into your life can have a profoundly positive impact on your mental wellbeing.

If you are buying this book to help someone else, by all means leave it lying around for them to see. But remember, the motivation has to come from them when they are ready.

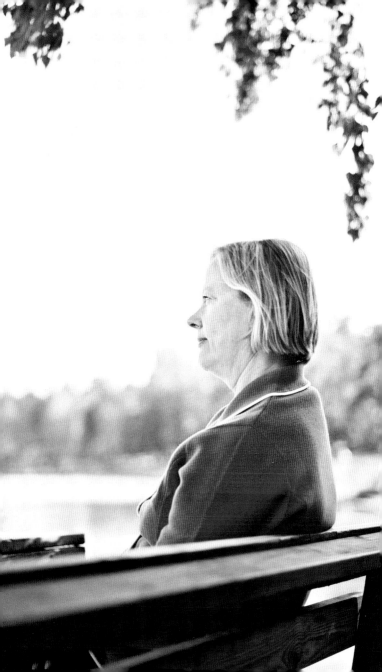

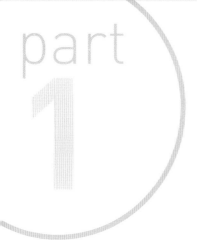

part

1

understanding depression

> > What is depression?

It is very normal to have ups and downs in our daily mood and most people feel blue from time to time. However when we feel down for more than two weeks it can develop into depression, a medical condition that can be diagnosed by a GP.

Different circumstances affect how people feel on a day-to-day (and sometimes minute-by-minute) basis: you may be looking forward to seeing a friend who then lets you down, or someone might criticise you at work. It is natural for our moods to change fairly often within a short space of time.

On the other hand, sometimes people feel down or depressed for more sustained periods of time. A house move might put you under immense pressure for several weeks, while the end of a relationship can leave you feeling unhappy for months, even years. Bereavement, unemployment, ill health, loneliness, low self-esteem, genetics, gender, family history, retirement – there are many factors that can affect a person's mental and physical wellbeing, and play a part in depression.

Sometimes we know that our low mood will pass: a new relationship or job will turn up, or our blues will simply melt away. But occasionally the low mood will persist, and this can be damaging.

Whatever the reason for it, the effects of depression are disabling for everyone, and some people find them so overwhelming that they consider harming themselves. That is why it's important to try and manage your mood. You can do this in a variety of ways: by consulting your GP, taking prescription medication if appropriate, or visiting a counsellor. You can identify the causes of your depression and, if possible, eliminate them.

And you can make some of the simple changes detailed in this book. A small step like adjusting your diet, tackling a bad habit or getting more active can really help. Getting through an episode using some of these techniques can make you stronger and more resilient, and help your regain control of your life.

> Depression is manageable. With the right steps most people can recover.

> ## WHAT ARE THE SYMPTOMS OF DEPRESSION?
Depression affects our whole way of being: how we think, feel and relate to others; our motivation to get through the day; our habits, behaviour and ability to feel pleasure; and how we cope with life in general.

Most people with depression will have at least five or six of the following symptoms:

- unhappy most of the time
- no interest in life
- difficulty making decisions
- can't cope anymore
- constant fatigue
- restlessness and agitation

- appetite loss or weight gain
- problems sleeping
- lack of sex drive
- no self-confidence
- feelings of inadequacy
- loneliness
- thoughts of self-harming

How common is depression?

Depression is very common, so no need to feel alone. In fact it is one of the most common psychological disorders treated by GPs, although even they sometimes have trouble spotting the symptoms. Have a look at these statistics:

- 20% of the population will experience some kind of mental health problem in the course of a year.
- Mixed anxiety and depression is the most common mental disorder in Britain.
- Depression affects 1 in 5 older people living in the community and 2 in 5 living in care homes.
- The UK has one of the highest rates of self-harm in Europe.
- 10–15% of women will receive a clinical diagnosis of post-natal depression (PND).
- One in 100 women will need to be hospitalised due to extreme PND.
- It is estimated that over 20% of people with serious depression never seek help from their GP.
- 40% of those who visit their GP with depression are not diagnosed, because they present themselves with another physical illness that masks their depression.

(www.rcpsych.ac.uk / Mental Health Foundation)

And depression is not a condition of the weak – far from it. Some famous people who have experienced depression include Sir Isaac Newton, Abraham Lincoln, Winston Churchill, Vincent Van Gogh, Ernest Hemingway, Spike Milligan, Tony Hancock and Bill Oddie.

> > What are the different types of depression?

Depression or 'low mood' can be a period of a few days or weeks when we experience a combination of the symptoms on pages 2 and 3. However there are specific terms for some other forms of depression listed below, some of which are long-lasting or recurring.

CLINICAL DEPRESSION

Clinical depression is a severe case of depression that has been diagnosed by a doctor. People with clinical depression lose their zest for life and the motivation to take care of themselves. It applies when a low mood is present for a minimum of two weeks and is combined with at least four of the following symptoms:

- Sleep problems – insomnia (not being able to sleep) or hypersomnia (sleeping all the time)
- Negative feelings – feeling helpless, worthless, guilty or hopeless
- Inability to focus and concentrate
- Lack of energy, no 'get up and go'
- Eating disturbances – loss of appetite or rapid weight gain
- Suicidal thoughts and desire to self-harm

Although a major depressive episode of this kind may occur just once, many people experience them repeatedly throughout their lives. Without treatment, the symptoms can last for months or years and suicide is a major risk. It is estimated that within five years of suffering a major episode, a quarter of sufferers will attempt to take their own lives.

BIPOLAR DISORDER OR MANIC DEPRESSION

Most people experience ups and downs in life. Bipolar disorder, or manic depression, is when the highs and lows are so extreme that they interfere with everyday activities and cause you to behave in uncharacteristic ways. About 1% of the adult population has bipolar disorder. It usually starts around adolescence and rarely after the age of 40.

Everyone's experience of bipolar disorder is different: some people have mainly lows with just the occasional period of mania, while others have a greater proportion of manic highs; for some the highs and lows are relatively brief, while for others they they may last for many months; some people have several episodes a year, some only a few in a lifetime.

The main treatments are drugs combined with therapy. The drugs are *mood stabilizers* such as lithium, which reduce the extreme swings in mood. Therapy can include being a part of a group, going on a course, or meeting with a nurse or occupational therapist. Both go hand in hand to help you manage your mood.

SEASONAL AFFECTIVE DISORDER (SAD)

SAD is probably one of the most common forms of depression with about 3% of the population suffering from it each year. It is thought that a lack of daylight affects the chemicals in the brain, which is why it occurs during the autumn and winter months, and tends to disappear during the spring and summer. Having said that, people who spend a lot of time indoors are also more likely to suffer from SAD.

Many of the symptoms are the same as those described on pages 2 and 3, and they are often worse in the morning. In non-seasonal depression, people sleep less and eat less; in SAD, they usually sleep *more* and eat *more*. If you have SAD, you may find it more difficult to wake up on a winter morning and can often feel sleepy during the day. You may crave sugary or high-carbohydrate foods, and since you probably won't be as active, it's easy to put on weight.

Seasonal affective disorder can be counteracted by a big dose of daylight. Many other forms of depression can also be treated to some extent simply by getting outside, or getting more active – and that is what this book is all about.

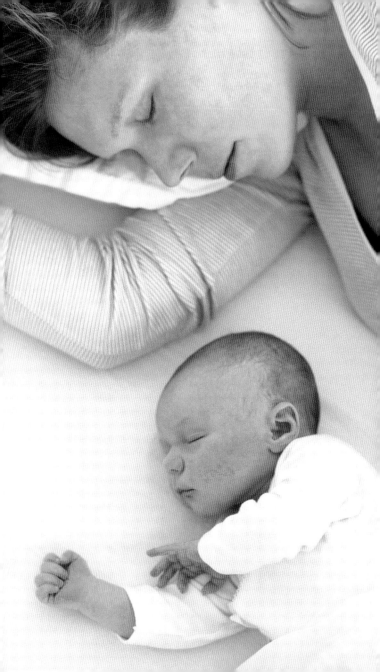

POST-NATAL DEPRESSION (PND)

About one in ten mothers will suffer with PND after having a baby. Most cases start within six months of giving birth, but it can develop up to two years later. PND can affect anyone, but women are more vulnerable if they do not have a partner, if their baby is born prematurely or is ill, if they are particularly stressed or have suffered from depression previously, or if they lost their own mothers at a young age.

The symptoms are similar to clinical depression. Women with PND often find themselves feeling guilty, irritable, anxious and tired; they can have problems sleeping, lose their appetites and their interest in sex, and generally feel they cannot cope.

PND can last for a few months or, more rarely, for years. Mild PND is usually helped with support from family and friends. More severe PND will require assistance from a health visitor or GP.

> > What causes depression?

Depression cannot always be explained. However there are some factors that are known to cause or contribute to depression, and these are looked at in more detail in this section.

Risk factors for depression

- Gender
- Genetic disposition
- Environmental and social factors
- Chemicals
- Early life experiences
- Self-worth
- Thinking patterns
- Repressed or suppressed emotions

> ### GENDER
Depression is generally reported to be more common in women than in men. However this may actually be the result of cultural and social constraints that cause men to mask or suppress their feelings more than women do.

> ### GENETIC DISPOSITION
We are more likely to experience depression if another family member has experienced it, but there is no evidence to indicate that a specific genetic link exists. It is possible that it happens because families occupy similar environments, share common ways of dealing with emotions and situations and learn behaviours and beliefs from each other.

> ### ENVIRONMENTAL AND SOCIAL FACTORS
Work stress, relationships, illness, bereavement, unemployment, having children, getting divorced … these are all factors that have the potential to cause depression, especially if the symptoms are not recognised and the condition dealt with.

> ### CHEMICALS
Inside your brain there are millions of cells that send and receive messages using chemicals called *neurotransmitters*. During depression, there is evidence to suggest that two of these neurotransmitters are affected more than others. These are called *serotonin* and *noradrenaline*.

Medication can help increase the concentration of these chemicals so that the messages in the brain can be transmitted efficiently, making you feel better. On the other hand, a poor diet or overuse of alcohol and drugs can lead to an imbalance in these chemicals.

> ### EARLY LIFE EXPERIENCES
Painful childhood experiences – being emotionally or physically abused, losing a loved one – can impact on our mental health as adults. A lack of attachment to a significant person during the early years can also cause long-term depression later in life.

This 'attachment theory' assumes that we are all social beings born with a need for intimate relationships. These intimate relationships start at birth, usually with our mothers (or a significant other like a grandparent). As a baby, we cry out for our needs to be met – in a healthy relationship, our mothers respond with the right amount of attention. From this secure base, we explore our world knowing that we can come back to our mother and be greeted with affection. An insecurely attached child can be very clingy, afraid to explore their world and angry with their mother. Research has now shown that this type of child quite often experiences mental ill-health repercussions later in life.

Having said this, most parents will do their best with the resources they have available. Attachment theory also suggests that there is no such thing as the ideal parent and that being 'good enough' should allow us to develop a healthy mental wellbeing.

> ## SELF-WORTH
People with chronically low self-esteem or self-worth are more at risk of depression than people who are at ease with themselves. There are many reasons why people develop low self-esteem. The crucial thing is to recognise that this is a contributing factor – only then can you begin to deal with it.

> ## THINKING PATTERNS
This is classic 'glass half empty' versus 'glass half full' territory. *This is terrible, I'm going to fail, what's the point* ... Constant negative thinking can force your mood to spiral down towards depression and keep you there. There are strategies to help people break out of negative thinking patterns once they have been identified, however.

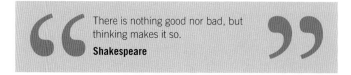

> There is nothing good nor bad, but thinking makes it so.
> **Shakespeare**

> ## REPRESSED OR SUPPRESSED EMOTIONS
It is also suggested that depression and low mood can be the result of feelings or emotions that are kept buried. These can sometimes explode

inappropriately, but can also remain hidden as a person goes about their daily tasks. In the long term, wearing a mask and pretending to be someone we are not causes a sense of incongruence inside of us, which is a common cause of mental-health problems.

>> How can depression be treated?

> Asking for help is not a sign of weakness or giving in – it is an essential resource.

The aim of this book is to show you some of the tools that you can use to help lift yourself out of depression. Part 2 focuses on mental approach and lifestyle, while Part 3 deals with being more active and taking exercise. These two approaches taken together can improve your mental wellbeing enormously, and for some readers may prove sufficient to beat back depression for good. However, for those with prolonged or very debilitating bouts of depression it's a good idea to look elsewhere for help at the same time.

> VISIT YOUR GP
The first line of treatment should always be to go to your GP and ask for their help. We would not hesitate to go to the doctor if we had flu, so why should we feel uncomfortable visiting the GP when we are mentally unwell? Depression has been referred to as the 'common cold of mental problems' (Seligman: 1998), and it's important to think of it as an illness. It can happen to anyone – Winston Churchill called depression his 'black dog' – and a person suffering from it is entitled to seek support and treatment.

Your GP may, after talking to you, decide to prescribe some medication. Most would recommend that medical treatment goes hand in hand with self-help strategies, and possibly therapy or counselling: it is really important to address the *cause* of depression, not just the symptoms. The strategies recommended will depend on the severity of the depression, and on individual circumstances.

I remember going to the GP when I was 17 because I was feeling 'not right': I had lost a lot of weight and my periods had stopped. I ended up crying in the surgery and I could not believe it – I hated crying. My doctor immediately put me on antidepressants. I didn't really know what they were at the time, and when they did not make me feel better I just took another one and another one.

I ended up collapsing at work and was sent to the hospital to have my stomach pumped. After this experience I was referred to a psychiatrist. It turned out that my depression was a reaction to a specific life experience; one I managed to address with their help. Many years later I trained as a counsellor so that I could help others. We are so much more open about mental health today, thank goodness, and there is much more support available – there's no need to suffer in silence.

Pat, aged 50

> **MEDICATION**

Research shows that after three months of treatment, 50% to 65% of individuals improve if given an antidepressant. However this approach should always go hand in hand with self-help, therapy or counselling, if the cause is to be treated as well as the symptoms, otherwise your depression is likely to return.

There are three main types of medication:

1. **SSRIs, or selective serotonin reuptake inhibitors:** these are commonly prescribed as they have fewer side effects than other medications.
2. **Tricyclic antidepressants:** these are prescribed less frequently because of adverse reactions with other drugs and more frequent side effects.
3. **MAOI, or monoamine oxidase inhibitors:** the reactions with other drugs and the side effects also mean this drug is prescribed less often.

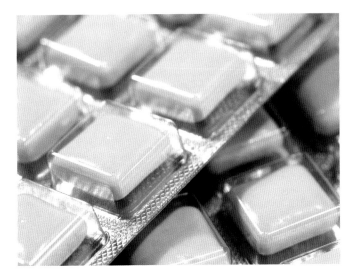

The side affects of these different types of medication are varied and include: dry mouth, fast heartbeat, constipation, sleepiness, weight gain, high blood pressure, nausea, indigestion and interference with sexual function. If you have been prescribed medication, check the leaflet that comes with it to see what the specific side effects are, and bear in mind that most of them wear off in a few days or weeks. If you are concerned, check with your GP.

Antidepressants are helpful but they won't treat the *cause* of your depression. It is always advisable to combine medication with an alternative approach such as counselling and exercise.

If you stop taking medication within eight or nine months the symptoms of depression are likely to return. The current recommendation is to continue with antidepressants for at least six months after you start to feel better. If you have two or more attacks of depression, treatment should be continued for at least two years. Meanwhile investigating the cause of your depression may help prevent a relapse in the long term.

Remember

If you are embarking upon a course of anti-depressants there are some important things to think about:

- Antidepressants should be monitored to make sure they are working effectively – keep in touch with your doctor, especially at the beginning.
- Your doctor may start you on a low dose then up your medication, so it is important to check in with your GP on a regular basis.
- It might be worth keeping a written record of your dose and how you are feeling – this is particularly useful if your doctor changes your prescription, and if you are trying different doses over a long period of time.
- You need to take them as they have been prescribed – if you skip days, they won't work.
- Give them a chance to work – they can take up to six weeks to have their full effect.
- Don't be put off by the side effects – they usually wear off in a few days.
- Persevere – stopping too early is the most common reason for a relapse. Even if you start to feel better, it is recommended that you keep taking antidepressants for at least six more months.
- Although antidepressants are not addictive, there can be some withdrawal symptoms when you stop taking them.
- Don't hesitate to contact your doctor if your side effects are severe or you are anxious, feeling worse or are tempted to take an overdose.

(Based on advice from the Royal College of Psychiatrists)

> ## TALKING TREATMENTS

Talking treatments can be very effective, particularly for people with mild to moderate depression. While some people find great comfort in talking to their family and friends about how they are feeling, others may feel they need someone with professional experience of depression, or prefer to go outside their immediate circle for support.

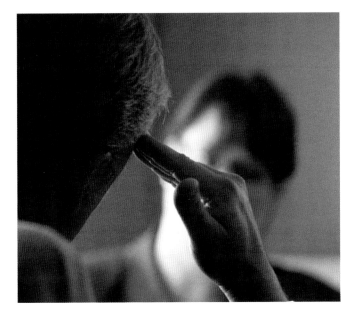

 It was several months before I realised I had depression. At first I thought it was fatigue from working too hard. Then I blamed the way I was feeling on other people, including my partner. It got to the point that I couldn't talk to anyone about how I was feeling. It was a lonely and difficult time.

So I finally took the plunge and went to see my doctor. She prescribed a course of antidepressants combined with regular counselling. The relief was immediate – I realised that I was just desperate to talk to someone. After a while I stopped needing the antidepressants, but the counselling itself remained an essential part of my recovery. It taught me the power of communicating and sharing how I feel, much to the relief of my friends and family. I know that I'll never allow my depression to isolate me like that again.

Alan, aged 44

When choosing a counsellor or therapist, you can start by visiting your GP – most surgeries have a counselling service available. Alternatively, check out the British Association for Counselling website (see the 'find out more' section at the back of the book) and ask them for a list of qualified counsellors in your area.

The key is to find a counsellor you like working with who offers an approach that suit your needs. You may have to do some research first, as there are many different styles of talking therapy and some of them might not work for you. Bear in mind that some of them will be free while others may be expensive. Consider also the time commitment required: is it a one-off treatment, or are they recommending a course lasting several weeks?

The list that follows gives a brief introduction to a range of talking treatments. You can find sources of further information in the 'find out more section' at the back.

COUNSELLING

Talking things through with a trained counsellor or therapist can be a relief – it can help you to clarify how you feel about your life and other people, and supports you as you work through your options. Your GP can usually arrange for you to be referred to a counsellor.

COGNITIVE BEHAVIOURAL THERAPY (CBT)

Many of us have set habits of thinking and acting. Sometimes these are negative and play a part in our depression. CBT helps break down the problem we are confronting into understandable parts such as thoughts, feelings, physical reactions and behaviour so that they can be analysed and understood. Having identified unhelpful ways of thinking, a trained therapist can then guide you as you develop a more realistic and positive approach.

Check with your GP or on the internet to see if there are any CBT therapists in your area and whether you can be referred. There may be a charge.

How does Cognitive Behavioural Therapy (CBT) work?

CBT will help you think through each issue in your life and turn it around, breaking down each area. A trained therapist will help you identify the patterns in your thoughts and reactions that are unhelpful. Then they will guide you, step by step, in the process of developing thoughts and reactions that are more positive. Small changes can have big results – you don't need to change your entire personality! For example, here is a different way to approach the problem of taking exercise in a class environment when you haven't done any for a while, and feel quite nervous about it:

Problem: You want to try a new exercise class.

Thoughts: 'People are going to look at me' or 'I'm not going to be able to do it right.'

Feelings: Scared, worried.

Physical reaction: Sweaty palms, faster breathing, feeling sick.

Action: You don't go to the exercise class.

Problem: You want to try a new exercise class.

Thoughts: 'I might meet new friends' or 'I will get to learn new exercises.'

Feelings: Scared, a little bit excited, hopeful.

Physical reaction: A slightly racing heart but no other symptoms.

Action: Go to the exercise class and enjoy it.

Next time you want to attend an exercise class, there will be less fear and avoidance as you build on the positive effect you have already achieved.

In summary, CBT helps you to:

- Identify any unrealistic and unhelpful ways of thinking
- Develop new, more helpful ways of thinking and behaving

RELATIONSHIP THERAPY

If your depression is connected to your personal relationships, the organisation Relate might help you. Relate specialise in working with relationships of any sort: spouse, partner, friends, family or work. The service is offered to singles and couples, either alone or with a partner, so you do not need to attend with the person whose relationship is troubling you. They also provide phone and on-line counselling, but there is a charge for this service.

SUPPORT GROUPS AND GROUP THERAPY

If there is a particular contributing factor to your depression you may be able to find a support group to help you deal with it. This applies to problems such as alcoholism and drug addiction, to many disabilities and long-term illnesses, and to people who are caring for someone with a disability or illness. There are many other kinds of support networks too, so it's always worth investigating to see if there's one suitable for you.

Support groups often involve sharing experiences and stories, and passing on tried and tested techniques for dealing with the problems their members are experiencing. They can help with things like benefits, medication and debt, and show you where to go to seek help. Although attending your first session can be daunting, there are huge advantages to sharing your problems and learning from other people. You can find out about support groups by looking online, visiting www.mind.org.uk or asking your GP.

BEREAVEMENT COUNSELLING

It can take a long time to recover from the death of someone close to you. The depression this causes is sometimes made worse by the fact that people 'don't like to talk about it' – you yourself may feel reluctant to share your feelings, or you may find that other people are awkward and prefer to avoid the subject. In this case you need to talk to a specialist bereavement counsellor: Cruse Bereavement Care is a helpful charity that offers advice and counselling.

INTERPERSONAL AND PSYCHODYNAMIC PSYCHOTHERAPY

This kind of treatment may be more suitable if you have had long-standing difficulties with your life or relationships. The therapist will help you to make connections between your past and present. This can help to show how some of the things that you feel, do and say are not driven by your conscious thoughts and feelings, but by unconscious feelings from your past. When you understand these connections better, you can make decisions based on what you want or need now, not on what your past experiences drive you to do.

> SELF-HELP AND COMPLEMENTARY THERAPIES

There is a wide range of other self-help ideas and complementary therapies that can be used to assist with treatment of low mood and depression. For example, yoga provides a combination of exercise and breathing focus that can be very beneficial for some people. Some of these techniques are covered in Part 2, but there are so many different resources and options that we could not cover them all here. Some will work for you and some won't – it depends on your personality and lifestyle. A little experimentation will be necessary to find the right one for you. Whatever you do, remember that a little goes a long way. One small step down the path towards helping yourself can have a very positive effect.

Here are some of our suggestions for ways to help yourself to a better mood:

- Exercising and physical activity
- Getting enough sleep
- Improving your diet and nutrition
- Drinking plenty of water
- Reducing caffeine and alcohol intake
- Using herbal remedies
- Quitting smoking
- Taking care of yourself
- Having some interests
- Developing your social life

- Focusing on improving your working life
- Managing your money
- Being more assertive
- Addressing your time management
- Thinking about your posture
- Having some recharging time
- Relaxation and meditation
- Acupuncture
- Spending time outdoors
- Growing something in your garden
- Making, building or restoring something

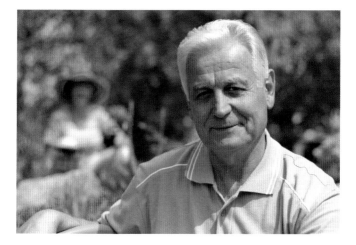

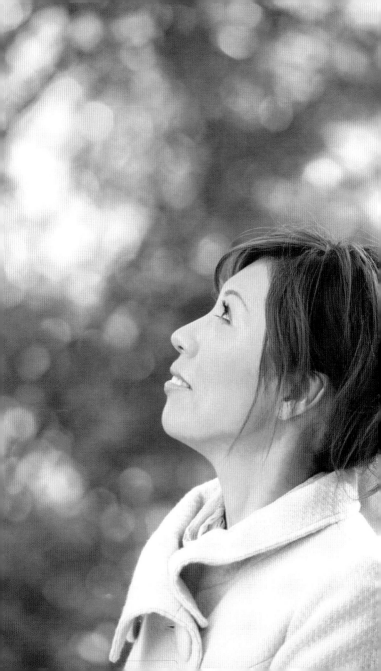

part

helping yourself
to health

In this part we will explore some self-help tools for making simple, positive changes to improve your mood. They can help you take back the responsibility (personal power) and take charge (personal control), so that you manage the depression rather than letting it control you. Then there is a brief lifestyle section, which is designed to give you plenty of ideas about how to improve your habits. At the very end there is a 'personal commitment table', where we hope you will want to record your new goals and your newfound sense of purpose.

The four-step strategy

There are four straightforward steps to making changes and taking control. We look at each of them in more detail later, but here is a brief sumnmary:

STEP 1: SELF-ASSESSMENT

Your starting point is to make an accurate assessment of your life. The simple table on page 26 is designed to help you examine different areas – for example diet, exercise, work, interests – and rate your level of satisfaction from 1 (poor) to 4 (good). This will show you the parts of your life that need attention. Don't worry if it seems to be a lot to do, you don't have to change them all at once.

STEP 2: SETTING GOALS

The next step is to set yourself some positive goals. Be realistic here: it may be that you have to compromise in some areas, for example if you are a new parent suffering from lack of sleep, if you're short-staffed at work, or going through a divorce. Try to identify only those areas that you can change and remember that even one small improvement can have a profound effect.

STEP 3: MAKING CHANGES

The third step is to put your changes into practice. Again, it's important not to try and do too much. This can lead to you feeling a sense of failure and abandoning the attempt early on. It's better to start with one small thing and do it well – then you'll feel inspired to move on to the next.

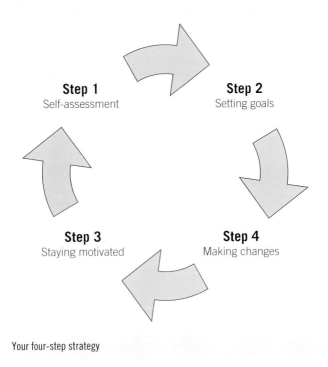

Step 1
Self-assessment

Step 2
Setting goals

Step 3
Staying motivated

Step 4
Making changes

Your four-step strategy

STEP 4: STAYING MOTIVATED

Think about ways to monitor and reward your progress. It can be hard to stay motivated at the best of times, and is particularly difficult when your mood is low. Learn to reward yourself for your achievements and put some thought into how you will manage any relapses.

We will look in more detail at each of these steps in the section that follows. Be ready to take an honest look at your life and habits – it might help to have a pen and paper to hand.

> For me, taking up a positive habit is far easier than giving up a negative habit. I was a heavy smoker for twenty years, even though I am asthmatic. I could feel the impact on my health, but my attempts at giving up always failed. I became demoralised and unhealthy, and thought I would always be limited by my smoking.
>
> Then a friend of mine suggested that instead of 'giving up' I should try 'taking up'. I decided to buy a bicycle and took up cycling the short distance to work. Soon I found that the good feeling the exercise gave me counteracted my craving for cigarettes. So as well as gaining the health benefits of exercise, cycling gave me a tool to beat my smoking for good.

Becky, aged 36

STEP 1: WHERE AM I NOW? SELF-ASSESSMENT

The table on page 26 is a simple way to assess eight aspects of your life and see which areas are unbalanced. Consider how you feel about each of them and rate them on a scale of 1 to 4. If in doubt, the questions on pages 24 and 25 should help you get started.

1 = lowest score indicating that you not satisfied with, or devote little time to, this aspect of your life
2 = not particularly happy with this aspect of your life
3 = fairly happy with this aspect of your life
4 = highest score indicating that you are very satisfied with, or devote lots of time to, this aspect of your life

Assessing your life

If you're unsure how to begin, ask yourself questions about each area of your life. Here is a guide to help you get started.

1. **Work:**
   - Is my work rewarding? Am I happy to remain in my role? *If yes, put 4.*
   - Do I find aspects of your work rewarding and enjoyable? *If yes, put 3.*
   - Is my work tolerable? *If yes, put 2.*
   - Do I hate going into work every day and often feel I just can't face it? *If yes, put 1.*

2. **Exercise:**
   - Am I active and do I exercise regularly (half an hour five times a week)? *If yes, put 4.*
   - Am I fairly active and do I take some regular exercise? *If yes, put 3.*
   - Am I fairly inactive, exercising sporadically? *If yes, put 2.*
   - No exercise at all? *Score this as 1.*

3. **Social:**
   - Do I make time for social activities every week? *If yes, put 4.*
   - Do I make some time for social activities but would like to do more? *If yes, put 3.*
   - Do I only very occasionally enjoy a social life? *If yes, put 2.*
   - Do I feel lonely and isolated? *If yes, put 1.*

4. **Health:**
   - Do I take good care of my health? *If yes, put 4.*
   - Do I have a healthy lifestyle most of the time with occasional lapses? *If yes, put 3.*
   - Do I drink too much / smoke quite often? *If yes, put 2.*
   - Do I drink too much / smoke on a regular basis? *If yes, put 1.*

5. **Diet:**
   - Do I have a healthy diet? *If yes, put 4.*
   - Do I have a healthy diet most of the time? *If yes, put 3.*
   - Do I eat healthily only now and then? *If yes, put 2.*
   - Do I neglect my diet and eat a lot of unhealthy foods?
     If yes, put 1.

6. **Interests and passions:**
   - Do I regularly enjoy hobbies or take part in something that
     interests me? *If yes, put 4.*
   - Do I pursue my interests on a fairly regular basis?
     If yes, put 3.
   - Do I only occasionally try to take part in something?
     If yes, put 2.
   - Do I miss out on hobbies and interests altogether?
     If yes, put 1.

7. **Sleep:**
   - Do I get a good night sleep every night? *If yes, put 4.*
   - Are my sleeping patterns occasionally disturbed?
     If yes, put 3.
   - Do I often have problems sleeping? *If yes, put 2.*
   - Do I have problems almost every night? *If yes, put 1.*

8. **Recharge time:**
   - Do I find time every day for myself? *If yes, put 4.*
   - Do I occasionally find time during the week to recharge?
     If yes, put 3.
   - Do I manage to find time only very infrequently?
     If yes, put 2.
   - Do I have no time for myself but spend most of it working or
     doing things for others? *If yes, put 1.*

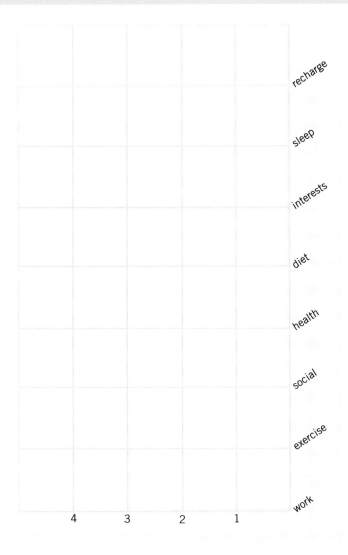

For each aspect mark your position with an X on the graph, then join up the Xs

STEP 2: WHAT WOULD I LIKE TO CHANGE? SETTING GOALS

Set yourself SMART goals

- **S**pecific: what exactly are you going to do?
- **M**easurable: how can you measure your target?
- **A**chievable: is it manageable for you?
- **R**ealistic: will you do it?
- **T**ime-framed: when, how often?

Once you have completed your graph, ask yourself the following questions:

1. **Which areas of my life are unbalanced?** There may be only one or two dips in your graph, or perhaps you have scored very low in all areas. Don't worry: you can take small steps to big results.

2. **What would I like my graph to look like?** Are there some areas of your life that you would like to score higher on and 'smooth your ride'? If so, place a cross to indicate where you would like to see these changes on your graph.

3. **Where do I start?** Again, it's important to be realistic. There may well be some things you cannot change. For example, if you are unhappy at work, it can take a long time to decide what to do about it and then put it into action. Or there may be too many things for you to change at once. So try to identify one area where you *can* focus on change: for example, most people are able to improve their diet and get more active.

STEP 3: HOW DO I TURN MY GOAL INTO ACTION?

It's great to say you want to eat more healthily, sleep better, exercise more … But how do you achieve this? Being specific is key. Breaking your goal down into small, easy-to-achieve steps makes it much more realistic and helps you get started. For example:

Goal: 'To take regular exercise' can be turned into a measurable target: 'to walk for 30 minutes on 5 days of this week'. This can be broken down further, so you goal becomes:

- I will walk for 10 minutes after each meal.

Goal: 'To relax more' can become a measurable target: 'I will relax for 15 minutes when I get home from work.' This can be made more achievable by breaking it down to:

- I will go straight to the garden with a book when I get home; no TV, no housework, just a few minutes of 'me' time.

Tip

Before you begin putting a goal into action, complete the personal commitment table on page 55. It will help you keep track of your goals and remind you why you are doing what you are doing. Read through the rest of this section first, though, for advice and guidance on improving your lifestyle.

It is also important to set a start date or time. You can always start next week, or tomorrow – but why not start right now? Making progress towards your goal has a very positive psychological effect, and will help you build up momentum.

STEP 4: HOW CAN I KEEP GOING? STAYING MOTIVATED

It is so easy to lose sight of all the positive steps you are taking and the changes you are making. For this reason, it's important to review your progress and notice everything that you do, rather than focusing on the things you don't. There is no need to feel downhearted if you miss an exercise session or if you eat the wrong food or have too much to drink. The key to making changes is to allow yourself to do it gradually.

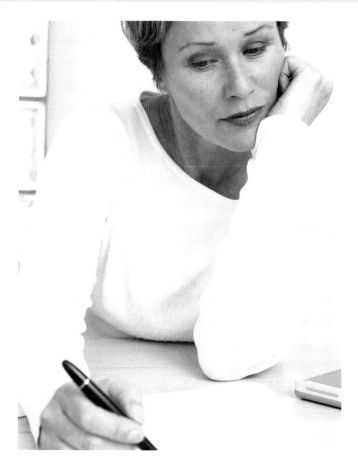

Write it down

It can really help to keep a record, focusing on the positive changes you make by recording them in a logbook. It is amazing how forgetful the mind can sometimes be about the positive things we do. You only have to think about the way one criticism can wipe out twenty compliments to realise the power of negative thinking. Depression can get us into a downward spiral and we forget to look in another direction. Reading back over the record of the efforts you actually have made is usually a pleasant surprise.

If you slip up and relapse a lot, perhaps you have set your goal too high and it is not realistic? In this case, go back and check that your goal is SMART for you (see page 27).

Know yourself

Occasional slips are a natural part of the process of change and we can learn from them. Get to know yourself: be a student of your life and identify the danger signs. If you get down and demoralised when you are over-tired, try to get enough sleep each night. If you eat when you are depressed, keep healthy snacks to hand. If you can't resist smoking socially, stay away from people who smoke, at least during the early days of giving up.

You can't always have a strategy to prevent slips though – learn to forgive yourself, and begin again. It is also important to remember that no one can keep up their good intentions at all times. If you do step off the straight and narrow, make sure you enjoy yourself while you're at it! Then afterwards remind yourself about the goals you set, and why, and carry on in a positive fame of mind.

Catch the unhelpful thought

Look out for the unhelpful and negative thoughts that decrease your motivation. Simply spotting them is very useful, allowing you to think before you give in to their negative influence.

Whenever you find yourself thinking or speaking a negative thought ('I am no good', 'I can't do this'), call time out or shout 'stop.' Recognise the thought for what it is, then just let it go.

This is a technique that takes time and practice, but it does get easier. It increases an awareness of your own thought patterns and helps you break free from negative cycles.

Mind your language

Notice the words you use to dictate your life experience. Use words that enable you take responsibility and be powerful, rather than words that disempower you and keep you low.

Don't use:

- I must
- I ought
- I can't
- I'll fail
- It's not my fault

Do use:

- I want
- I choose
- I can
- I'll learn
- I can handle this

For example, change 'I must exercise today' to 'I want to exercise today'. It's your right to choose: you can.

On the road to taking control

Steve Jonas in ACSM's *Exercise is Medicine* (2009) suggests that having the motivation to make changes and then mobilising that motivation are the central factors to lifestyle change. He defines motivation as 'the mental process that connects a thought or a feeling with an action.'

To make changes and stay motivated we have to 'take control' and 'take responsibility'. By thinking about the four-step strategy and completing the graph on page 26, you have already begun this process. You have made the first steps towards taking control and responsibility – an excellent start.

Now you've reached the end of this section, read through the lifestyle focus that follows. There is plenty of information to help you change areas of your life for the better, from getting a good night's sleep to managing stress. Once you've read through this section, turn to the personal commitment table on page 55. You don't have to fill it in if you don't want to, but it is a useful tool to remind you where you're going, and why.

Lifestyle focus

The greatest changes you can make to improve your overall health and combat depression are simple yet effective. From taking time to focus on your breathing (page 51) to exercising for half an hour a day, there are lots of techniques to help you combat your low mood.

We will talk about exercise in detail in Part 3, but there are many other ways to change your lifestyle for the better. All of them play an important part in reducing the effects of depression.

GET ACTIVE

For some people the idea of exercise can seem daunting. However, introducing more physical activity into your day-to-day life can play a significant role in lifting your mood, managing depression and promoting good health. Whether you have long-term clinical depression or feel low every now and then, being active can help your efforts to take control.

The good news for those who don't feel ready or don't have time to start exercising is that physical activity doesn't have to involve going to a gym or an exercise class: it can be as simple as doing some weeding in your garden or hoovering the carpet. Increasing activity in these everyday areas can form a bridge to exercise for its own sake (with the added benefit of improving the appearance of your garden or carpet!)

It's easy to be active

Many of us lead sedentary lives, both at home and at work. The way we travel, work and socialise often involves sitting down, and all the energy-saving devices in our homes make us less active too.

But it's so easy to bring a little more activity into our day-to-day lives – and it's really beneficial too. Walk up the stairs instead of taking the lift; take a stroll in your lunch break; or walk to the shops instead of travelling by car or public transport. These simple goals can help make fresh air and exercise a regular part of your life. And you don't even have to join a gym.

The following three suggestions show you how easy and 'every day' being more active can be. Why not try:

1. **Going for a walk:** Walking is one of the best activities you can do. It involves being out of doors, which is beneficial for everyone and particularly those suffering from a seasonal form of depression. If you are walking in company you should walk at a rate where you can hold a conversation comfortably. If walking on your own, try to maintain a level where you feel warm but not completely out of breath.

2. **Cleaning the car:** This can be quite a vigorous activity with lots of bending and large movements from your arms and legs. Ideally, your breathing will have increased and you'll be feeling warm and sweaty – good signs!

3. **Climbing the stairs:** This is an activity that uses some of the largest muscles in the body. When climbing stairs (especially if it is more than a couple of flights), you will probably feel very out of breath and your leg muscles will tire quickly.

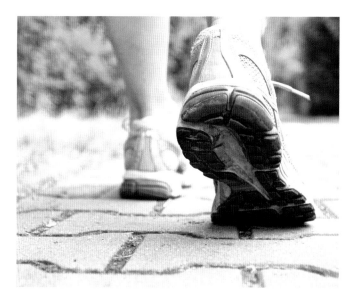

Not very fit?

If you are not used to being active or have a health issue that worries you, turn to the table on page 61 and see whether you're ready to get active. Also read the advice on how often to exercise on page 63, and what intensity to exercise at your page 64. Remember to start gently if you are in doubt, and build up to more sustained periods of activity or exercise as you grow more confident.

Other ideas for getting more active:

- Walk the dog
- Walk the kids to school
- Walk to the shops
- Walk in your lunch hour
- Do the shopping for your neighbour
- Exercise at your desk
- Do some gardening
- Do the housework with vigour
- Walk up escalators
- Put on some music and move around
- Park your car further away from the office or supermarket
- Buy a Wii Fit or an exercise video
- Join a walking group like the Ramblers
- Get on the bus a stop later or get off a stop earlier
- Take a detour round the park
- Learn bowling or badminton
- Walk home from the pub or restaurant

When I was at school I had to play netball every week. I was very little and not very co-ordinated and I was always the last to get picked for any team.

I gave up on exercise after that and really hated being forced to do anything active. Then one day my friend coaxed me out for a walk through the park at lunchtime. It relaxed me almost at once as we talked, breathing deeply and admiring the autumn leaves which I hadn't really noticed before.

Now I go to the park for a walk every day. It clears my mind and helps me tackle the afternoon with a better spirit. Although I still don't take part in any sports, I feel fitter and stronger and less hostile to the idea of exercise. So who knows, maybe I'll join a netball team one day?

Hilary, aged 31

> ## SLEEP

Depression can disrupt the sleeping cycle, either making you extremely sleepy or preventing you from sleeping. A lack of sleep will reduce your concentration and you will find it much harder to make decisions.

Going without sleep for 24 hours or getting only five hours sleep a night for a week is the equivalent of a blood alcohol level of 0.1%. This is the same as consuming four drinks for an average-sized person. The legal limit for driving in the UK is 0.08%, so you can see that a lack of sleep can make you act as if you are slightly drunk and have a big impact on your life.

It's not always easy to take control of a sleeping pattern that has been disrupted through depression. The tips and techniques below should assist you, but it's important to give yourself time – habits don't change overnight.

- Make sure your bedroom is at a comfortable temperature
- Get blackout blinds if it's too light
- If you can't sleep, get up and do something relaxing like reading or listening to music – don't lie there feeling frustrated
- Keep to regular sleeping times: try to get to bed at the same time every night, and get up at a sensible time too
- Have a relaxing bath to help you to unwind before you go to bed: water provides a comforting sensation for the body
- Set the mood: use candlelight or music to soothe you before sleeping

- Make sure your mattress is comfy and supports you well, and change it every 10 years or so
- Keep a notebook by your bed so that you can write down any thoughts that disrupt your sleeping patterns
- Keep the bedroom for sleeping, rather than watching television or other activities
- Try some meditation before you go to bed
- Listen to a relaxation tape or audiobook when you go to bed to help you drift off to sleep
- Take regular exercise, but don't exercise too close to bedtime
- Don't sleep during the day
- Don't drink coffee, alcohol or other stimulants before you go to bed
- Don't smoke before bedtime
- Don't eat your last meal close to bedtime
- Use a sleep log to record your sleeping patterns – it may be better than you think and therefore easier to manage

> I was having trouble sleeping because I was feeling really stressed and miserable. I tried keeping a notebook, but that didn't work for me – I can fill a whole book with my thoughts. So I invested in some audio books and put them on when I am going to be bed. My mind can wander off at times, but the story brings me back and relaxes me. Soon enough I drift off and the only problem is that sometimes I never learn the end of the story!

Harry, aged 55

DIET

Food affects people in complex ways. It can give great pleasure or it can be used as a coping mechanism – something that brings its own problems. There is a lot of information about health and nutrition available, and we have all been told time and again about the importance of drinking plenty of water and getting our 'five a day' – five different portions of fresh fruit and vegetables each and every day. But taking control of our diet can play a significant part in improving our mental wellbeing as well as our physical health, and so it's worth looking again at the basics.

Food for thought

The chemicals in the brain that influence mood can be affected by the foods we eat. Many foods (especially processed) contain artificial chemicals, which can cause our body to react in different ways and affect our mood. Low levels of vitamins, minerals and essential fatty acids can also affect mental health: for instance, low levels of omega-3 oils (found in oily fish like sardines) have been linked to depression.

The charity Mind offers a wonderful guide to food and mood (see the 'find out more' section). Mind found that from a survey of 200 people, 88% reported that changing their diet for the better improved their feeling of wellbeing. In addition:

- 26% stated large improvements in mood swings
- 26% stated improvements in managing panic attacks and anxiety
- 24% stated improvements in their depression

Most of those surveyed said that cutting down on food 'stressors' and increasing the amount of food 'supporters' had a beneficial effect on their mood. This may be their subjective experience, and some might consider this the placebo effect. But for whatever reason, it seems to be true that eating more healthily does have the potential to influence your mood.

Stressor foods include: sugar, caffeine, dairy, alcohol, chocolate, processed food and food containing a large number of additives and saturated fats.

Supporter foods include: water, vegetables, fruit, nuts, seeds, fibre, wholegrain foods and oil-rich fish.

Everyone benefits from a balanced diet, meaning a diet that contains the right balance of all major food groups. The food pyramid below shows the proportion of each food type that should be eaten. The main, lower level of the pyramid is made up of fresh fruit and vegetables, and these should constitute the majority of your diet. The foods at the top – cake, biscuits, chocolate and so on – should make up only a tiny proportion of your daily diet.

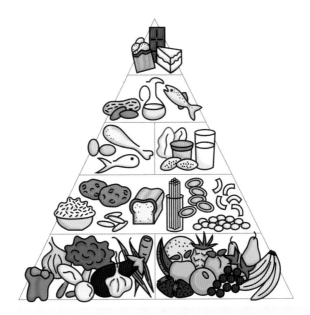

The food pyramid

Some additional steps you can take to improve your diet are:

- Eating regularly and not skipping breakfast.
- Eating more complex carbohydrates such as brown rice or wholemeal bread. Complex carbohydrates are a primary source of fuel for our body and can increase serotonin levels in the brain, which help to improve our mood.

- Eating less saturated fat. It can make us feel unhealthy and demoralised if we eat too much fatty food. Too much also increases the risk of high cholesterol and furring of the artery walls, which puts us at risk of other diseases, such as high blood pressure and coronary heart disease.
- Eating less sugar and salt.
- Eating sufficient fibre.
- Eating more fruit and vegetables (at least five a day).
- Balancing your calorie intake. Too few calories will slow down the metabolism and make you feel lethargic; too many calories will be stored as body fat and cause weight gain.
- Drinking more water. People often mix up feelings of hunger with thirst. If you are overweight, try taking a glass of water or fruit tea and see if you still feel hungry.
- Eating only when you feel hungry.

Tip

It takes about 20 minutes for our brain to register when we have eaten enough. This means that you can carry on eating for 20 minutes after you're full without realising. Try to eat more slowly and wait a while before having that second helping to see if you really want it.

FANCY A TIPPLE?

Drinking too much can increase the risk of liver damage, cirrhosis of the liver and cancer of the mouth and throat. But did you know that alcohol is also a depressant? It may initially have a lifting affect on the mood, but the after-effects of drinking short-term – and the long-term effects of alcohol misuse – are well documented. The long and the short of it is that drinking too much is bad for us physically, and definitely unhelpful when dealing with depression.

It is all too easy to develop a drinking habit, especially if used to escape the stresses and difficulties of life. Many people drink a bit too much – it is a shortcut to feeling relaxed. But it's all too easy to slip into an addictive cycle. For some people, cutting down on excess alcohol consumption can make the symptoms of depression miraculously disappear. But how much is too much?

It's worth noting that the amount of alcohol contained in pub measures such as a pint or glass of wine has increased over the years. An average bottle of wine used to be 9% alcohol by volume (ABV) with 6 units in a bottle but nowadays it is more likely to be 13.5% or higher and contain at least 10 units. The same applies to beers and spirits. This means that many of us may be unwittingly drinking much more than we should be.

Binge drinking is also increasingly common. This usually happens in a social environment and therefore seems acceptable, but it can be a way of masking a serious problem. A 'binge' is drinking more than twice the recommended daily amount in one session: for women this would be six units in an evening (or two large glasses of wine in the pub), and for men it would be eight units.

Maximum recommended units of alcohol		
	Units of alcohol	
Health risk	*Women*	*Men*
☺ No significant risk	2–3 units per day (no more than 14 per week)	3–4 units per day (no more than 21 units per week)
☹ Increasing risk	3 or more units per day on a regular basis	4 or more units per day on a regular basis

" I was used to going out on the town with my friends at weekends. Then I started a new job and began drinking with work colleagues during the week too. The trouble was, I drank as much on Monday as on Saturday. Before long I was suffering from intense anxiety that was beginning to tip towards depression. Everyone was worried about me and my doctor suggested antidepressants. Instead I cut back on my drinking, and after a while I felt much better. I still go to the pub with friends but I drink soft drinks and water as well as beer. It was a revelation to me that you can have fun without getting drunk. "

Amanda, aged 23

Units of alcohol in popular drinks

Measure/drink		Alcohol by volume	Units
Half pint of ordinary beer, lager or cider		4%	1.1
330ml bottle of strong beer		5%	1.7
Small glass of wine (125 ml)		12–14%	1.5–1.75
Large glass of wine (175 ml)		12–14%	2.1–2.45
Single measure of spirits		40%	1

It is recommended that alcohol should not be combined with some medications. There is a wealth of support out there if you are concerned with your drinking and we recommend you seek professional help. (See 'find out more' for details of information and support services.)

> ### A MORNING JOLT

Caffeine can have a negative effect on our mood too, so it's worth having a look at your daily intake. A low to moderate intake of caffeine is 130–300mg per day. To find out if you're within this limit, look at the table below. It may surprise you to see that five strong cups of tea takes you over the limit.

Caffeine content of popular drinks	
Product	**Caffeine (mg)**
Coffee	
Instant, weak (1 level tsp)	45
Instant, strong (1 heaped tsp)	90
Brewed, percolated, 20ml	100
Filtered, 200ml	140
Espresso (short black), 100ml	80
Cappuccino, 1 cup, 200ml	80
Tea	
Bag or brewed, weak, 200ml	20
Bag or brewed, strong, 200ml	70
Soft drinks	
Coke, 375ml	50
Pepsi, 375ml	38
Red Bull energy drink, 1 can, 250ml	80
Chocolate	
Dark, 50g	33
Milk, 50g	12

(Adapted from: Choice Health Reader, Jan/Feb 2001)

If you are consuming over 300mg a day it might be helpful to cut back, especially if you are struggling with disrupted sleep on anxiety. To reduce these negative symptoms try decaffeinated drinks, or simply drink more water: it offers the body more hydration and is both refreshing and healthy.

Herbal remedies for depression

Always check with your GP first before trying any of the following for depression. They all have potential problems with others drugs you may be taking – *always read the labels!*

- **St John's wort** (*hypericum perforatum*) – increases the neurotransmitter serotonin in the brain but can reduce the effectiveness of the contraceptive pill, and may also increase sensitivity to sunlight.
- **S-adenosyl-methionine** – helps to produce more neurotransmitters in the brain, with fewer side effects.
- **Folic acid (folate)** – helps to produce more neurotransmitters in the brain.
- **Selenium** – may prevent cell damage and produce the thyroid hormone.
- **Omega-3 fatty acids** – unknown as to how these work, but often used in conjunction with antidepressants.

THE EVIL WEED

The negative consequences of cigarette smoking on health are well documented. Carbon monoxide and nicotine are the two chemicals in cigarettes that have the most impact on the heart. Carbon monoxide contributes to decreased oxygen being circulated around the body to the tissues. Nicotine stimulates the production of adrenaline, which increases heart rate and blood pressure, causing the heart to work harder. Smoking also damages the lining of the coronary arteries and contributes to atherosclerosis, a build-up of fatty tissue on the artery walls. The tar in cigarettes causes cancer.

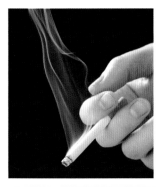

Smoking is highly addictive and once started it isn't easy to quit. If you want to stop smoking, contact a local smoking cessation group via your GP surgery to receive advice and support while you quit. (See 'find out more' for details of some information services.) Some people try to give up 100 times before they succeed. So never give up trying to give up – you can do it!

Even if you're not worried about the specific health concerns associated with smoking, bear in mind that it also has an impact on your mood. In particular, it can stop you from being active and taking exercise – both of which are important steps towards combating the effects of depression.

Habits

Sometimes it helps to replace a bad habit with something else, rather than leaving that 'empty hole' feeling. Some tips for replacing unhealthy habits with healthier habits are:

- Eat a piece of fruit
- Drink a glass of water if you feel hungry – often you're actually just thirsty
- Go for a short walk when you get tired – surprisingly, the exercise will actually refresh you
- Meditate or relax for five minutes at the start and end of each day
- Perform some short desk-relief exercises
- Go to an exercise session or join a walking group
- Drink a glass of water before you have that glass of wine
- Swap a cup of coffee for a herbal tea
- Move around the house before you sit to watch TV
- Do some breathing exercises before you have a cigarette

INTERESTS AND SOCIAL ACTIVITY

Those who are introverted by nature enjoy more time alone; those who are extroverted enjoy lots of company. Either way, we need to be taken out of ourselves on occasion, focussing on something external, whether it is a social activity or a solitary pursuit.

You might not think you have the time, energy, money or motivation to get involved with something new. However, hobbies don't have to be expensive, and having a leisure activity can be very helpful to your mood. You can also have fun if you share this interest with others.

If you want to develop your circle of social contacts it is useful to join a group where you can meet people. This may be an exercise class, a walking group or a course of some kind – learning Spanish or cookery for example. Meeting people is the first step towards developing friendships and building a social support network. Having a strong social support network can help you to make changes to your life and will provide motivation and encouragement. If you feel very shy at meeting new people, pick something that you feel will suit you or try catching up with someone who you haven't heard from in a while. You can also enjoy keeping in touch on the internet through email or a social networking site.

The way of overcoming shyness is to make small steps to chat to people and, as Susan Jeffers suggests in her book *Feel the Fear and Do It Anyway*, start expanding your comfort zone so that it grows bigger. Of course, not everyone will want to make conversation or be our friend (and vice versa) – this is natural. But to make more friends you

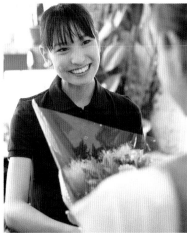

need to start networking and being a 'friend'. You don't have to suddenly walk into a crowded club and start socialising – you can start by talking to the checkout staff at a local supermarket or saying hello to your neighbours. And if someone speaks to you, answer them.

> > Managing stress

Stress, whether it's at home or at work, can develop into long-term depression. Many people experience stress at work, and for lots of different reasons. We may not like the work we do. We may not feel fulfilled by our job, or we may experience difficulty in our relationships. Being too busy – or even not being busy enough – often causes stress.

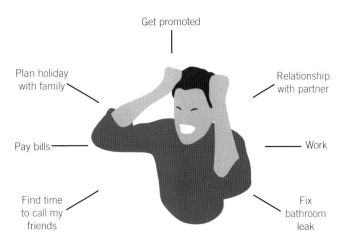

Get promoted

Plan holiday with family

Relationship with partner

Pay bills

Work

Find time to call my friends

Fix bathroom leak

Remember that the things you do throughout the day will have an impact on your stress levels, both at home and at work. Smoking and drinking too much may help in the short term, but ultimately they will affect your health and increase your stress levels. On the other hand, taking ten minutes a day to perform some desk-based exercises will improve your mood (see page 69). Even just simply being aware of your posture and sitting correctly throughout your working day will really help alleviate some of the build-up of tension (see page 65).

It's important to analyse your life and identify areas where you feel stressed and out of control – and from there, take simple steps to regain control. Here are a few tips to help you:

1. Be assertive

Being assertive is about respecting who you are while at the same time respecting others. Sometimes your wants and needs match those of other people and sometimes they don't, which can lead to disharmony. Sometimes we need to agree to disagree in relationships – and that is OK. The aim of assertiveness is to create a situation where everyone wins rather than one person winning at the expense of another.

We **all** have the right to:

- Ask for what we want
- Say: 'No'
- Have and express our own opinions, feelings and thoughts
- Make our own decisions and manage the consequences
- Change our minds
- Have time for ourselves
- Be successful
- Not know about something
- Choose whether to get involved with the problems of another
- Make mistakes
- Say: 'I don't understand'
- Be treated with respect
- Act assertively
- Choose not to assert ourselves

(Adapted from: Bayne et al. (1998:7), *The Counsellors Handbook*)

Becoming more assertive takes time and practise – you need to believe what you are saying in order to appear in control and this is not easy for some. However, the following steps are useful to help you take back control:

- Decide want you want
- State what you want clearly and specifically
- Use positive and confident language
- Relax and use positive body language
- Listen to the other person

- Stay focused
- Aim for a win–win situation
- Manage and respect your feelings

If you struggle to be assertive or if you feel that experiences in your present are triggering feelings from your past, it is wise to consider counselling, working through these issues in a supportive and non-judgmental environment. This will help you to develop greater self-awareness and build your own assertiveness.

> I really struggled to say no to any request a friend or family member made and I ended up running around trying to cram too much into my day and 'burning myself out'. I just got so low and then I would end up snapping at everyone and blaming them for being so demanding.
>
> A woman at one of the walking groups I go to told me that she used to always say yes to everyone and that she had attended a local assertiveness class. So I thought, well, if she can do it so can I and I enrolled! I learned so much – mainly that it isn't other people's fault if I cannot say no, nor is it mine. I learned that I had a choice. I could say no if I didn't want to do something or if I didn't have time, without having to give various excuses or reasons. It took lots of practice, and it still does, but it has helped me!

Pat, aged 51

2. Manage your time

Top tips for managing your time:

- **Write a list:** Whether it's at work or at home, make a list of things that need to get done, with the most urgent or important at the top. Tackle the things that you hate doing first so that they get done and don't get overlooked or carried over onto the list for the next day. For example do the accounts before you plan your business trip. At home do the housework before you do the gardening.

- **Prioritise:** Identify the important things and allocate time to them. Don't get caught spending lots of time on things that are not priorities. It is amazing how often people do this, even when they are so busy they are suffering from chronic stress.

- **Tackle one task at a time:** Set an achievable time frame (see the SMART goals on page 27) and reward yourself when you have finished. Hate cleaning the bathroom? Promise yourself a long soak in the clean and fresh tub afterwards, then tackle the next task.

- **Get 'chunky':** Break large or unpleasant tasks into smaller chunks to make them easier to tackle. For example, if you don't like doing your accounts, start by getting all your receipts together. Then put them in date order and input them onto a spreadsheet. Next tackle your income and so on. It make take you a few days but, as each chunk is shorter than the whole task, it will be much less stressful to do.

- **Remove interruptions:** Use answer-phones, 'do not disturb' signs on the door and check your emails at set times to avoid being distracted. Set your work phone to switch off at 8 p.m. and back on at 8 a.m. so you are not tempted to look at it or carry on working during your home time.

- **Be realistic:** We can't all be perfect at everything and most people struggle with balance in their lives. If you are a student, retired or

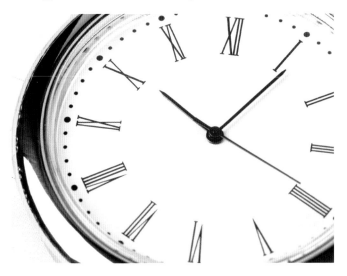

running a busy household it can be very difficult to manage the many conflicting demands on your time, and many workers find it impossible to fit all their chores and activities into evenings and weekends. Despite this pressure, it is vital to make some time for yourself.

- **Stick to a routine:** Plan your time and you'll be amazed at how much more you can get done – leaving you more 'me' time.
- **Pace yourself:** Save the activities that you love doing for your tired moments as these will lift your mood.
- **Say no firmly but politely:** Only take on what you can handle – there is usually someone who may have more time or be just as good at the task, so suggest them for the job.
- **Schedule regular breaks for meals and water:** Don't skip breakfast and do keep healthy snacks on hand for the sugar crashes. Skipping meals when under pressure only makes things worse.
- **Pay other people:** If you can afford to, employ a cleaner or gardener or get a babysitter or childminder in to give you some free time.

3. Having some recharging time

Ancient cultures often talk about our 'body, mind and spirit'. How often do we take time to nurture our 'spirit'? How often do we give out to others, but not put anything back into ourselves?

Making time for yourself – booking time in your diary if need be – is essential for maintaining a healthy life balance. It allows you to recharge your batteries. It's amazing how much better you feel when tackling a stressful situation if you've given yourself a break first.

Tip

If something is on your mind – whether it is work, personal or social – take a little time out. Walk for half an hour, or do ten minutes of exercises. When you return to your task or worry, you will find yourself feeling much more positive. A solution to a dilemma is far more likely to present itself.

Other things to try during your 'recharging' time:

- Write a list of all the things that are good about your life
- Indulge in a creature comfort and be kind to yourself
- Focus on your breathing
- Give yourself half an hour for exercise, relaxation or meditation
- Take yourself to a gallery, museum or cafe.

4. Focus on your breathing

One of the greatest gifts of life that we take for granted is our breath – our life force. Being aware of our breathing can help to distract our mind away from any low mood. Correct breathing enables us to take more oxygen into the lungs and can help to improve the posture of the upper spine and maintain mobility in this area. A few deep breaths when feeling stressed can really help, and its a technique that can be used anywhere, anytime with great results.

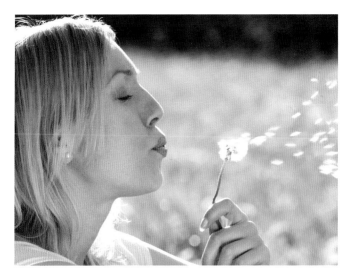

Breathing exercise

1. Start by finding an open, relaxed position – seated, lying or standing
2. Focus awareness on the depth, speed and feeling of your breathing
3. Close your eyes or focus on a specific spot looking forwards or slightly downwards (make sure your posture doesn't change)
4. Take the breath slightly deeper into the lower rib cage (most people take very shallow breaths into the upper chest area only)
5. Keep the breath soft, smooth and rhythmical
6. Find a natural breathing pace and power (not forcing or straining)
7. Let the breath become effortless and allow it to flow freely
8. Notice your abdomen rise and fall
9. Allow your lower rib cage to expand sideways (you can place your hands around the ribs if it helps)
10. Allow a few minutes just to focus on the breathing and stillness

5. Benson method of relaxation

Dr Herbert Benson used this method of relaxation to treat patients with high blood pressure. He suggested that individuals sit still and quietly focus on their breathing and, on every outward breath, say out loud the word 'one'.

Adapted version of the Benson method relaxation script:

- Sit quietly with an open body posture
- Focus on your breathing
- As you breathe out, focus on a desired word or mantra
- The word chosen can be spoken out loud or quietly to yourself
- Practise this for about 5–10 minutes, allowing the body to relax.

6. Meditation

Meditation is a great way of relaxing your mind and refreshing yourself.
Take time to sit quietly and let any unwanted or distracting thoughts
pass by and focus on your breathing and stillness.

A treat for your overworked mind

- Sit comfortably, back straight and supported, shoulders relaxed
  and arms resting gently
- Close your eyes
- Focus on breathing deeply and slowly for 10 counts
- Become aware of the activity of the mind and the speed of your
  thoughts
- Let the thoughts pass through the mind – let them go
- Focus on stillness
- Allow the mind to slow down
- Allow the mind to become quiet and silent
- Let go of other thoughts, acknowledge them, then release them
- Keep your focus on stillness
- Keep your focus on breathing
- Allow the mind to rest
- Allow the mind to be free and peaceful

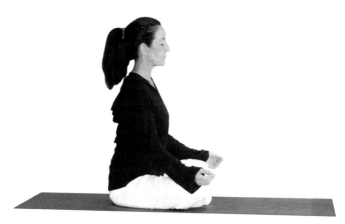

7. Be good to yourself

Make regular time for some creature comforts and things that make you feel good. Here are some suggestions:

- Bubble bath in candlelight with soft music
- Writing a letter to a friend or telephoning a friend
- Massage and aromatherapy
- Hot shower
- Curling up on the sofa with a video
- Sofa and a face pack
- Manicure and pedicure
- Horse riding in the countryside
- Day at a health spa
- Watching a feel-good film
- Dancing to a piece of music
- Making love with my partner
- Daydreaming anywhere peaceful, letting my thoughts come and go, and fantasising
- Visualising the gardens at a country retreat I visit
- Cuddling up with my teddy and letting myself feel sorry for myself
- Going for a walk with my daughter
- Listening to music by candlelight
- Sleeping
- Drawing pictures
- Going to the gym
- Booking a break so I have something to look forward to
- Drinking a cup of hot chocolate
- Driving to a place with great views – no cars, no people, no phones
- Walking my dog with a flask of tea and snacks
- Going for a run
- Cooking myself a special, healthy and nourishing meal

Note: Thanks to all the wonderful people who contributed their personal creature comforts to develop this list.

My personal commitment

I want to find more balance in this aspect of my life:

Choose the area where you would like to make changes.

More balance in this area would give me:

Express this by stating how you think addressing this area of your life would affect you – how you think, feel, behave; your health, etc.

I already have:

State a strength, achievement or interest in this area to remind you why you have chosen it.

My major goal for myself in this area of my life is:

Use the SMART strategy to determine this goal.

I want to achieve this by:

Write the date you would like to achieve this by – make sure it is realistic.

Three things I can do to move this area into balance are:

1

2

3

One action step I can take today is:

Start now! Identify one thing you can do today to help move you towards more balance in your life. *Any* action you take will count!

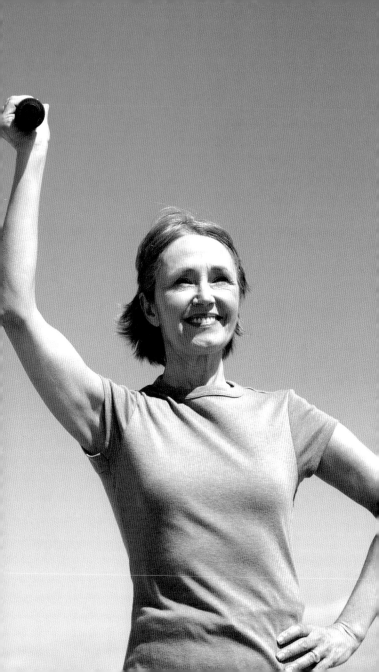

part

the exercises

> Exercise and you

Our body is designed to move: the skeleton is made up of many joints that enable us to move in lots of different directions and muscles that grow stronger with use. If we don't use the body, we lose some of the potential to move it and become stiff and immobile. This creates physical tension and a build-up of stress, and can contribute to some of the modern-day diseases that are linked to inactivity, such as obesity, arthritis, osteoporosis, diabetes, high blood pressure and coronary heart disease, as well as to depression.

Some of the physical benefits of exercise and being more active on a regular basis:

- Increases the strength of our heart
- Improves the circulation of blood and oxygen
- Improves the rate at which we breathe
- Improves the tone and strength of our muscles
- Improves the strength of our bones
- Lowers our blood cholesterol levels
- Lowers our blood pressure
- Burns calories and helps us to manage our weight

WHY IS EXERCISE IMPORTANT TO MANAGE OUR MOOD?

Most of us know that exercise is good for us and that once we get moving, we start feeling some of the benefits almost immediately. One of the positive side effects can be simply that we have some valuable time for ourselves.

The problem is that depression has a way of taking over your life, depleting both your mental and physical energy levels. However, if you want to make improvements to your mood and your health, it really is worth giving exercise and activity a go.

Regular exercise – whether at home, outside, in the pool or taking an exercise class – has a positive impact on our mental wellbeing in a number of ways:

- **Hormones/body chemicals:** Physical activity increases levels of the body's 'natural' mood enhancing chemicals (endorphins, serotonin and noradrenaline). These can be significantly reduced when we are feeling low or depressed, but exercise will stimulate their release, which explains the 'feel-good factor' we experience when we finally make our mind up to get more active.
- **Temperature:** Exercise and activity increase the circulation of blood, which in turn raises our body temperature. This helps to reduce muscle tension and increases our mobility. Feeling warm and more mobile can help to improve our mood.
- **Improved body image:** Regular exercise will improve our muscle tone and posture and can contribute to us feeling better about our body. We believe we look better, so we feel better.
- **Improved sleep:** Exercise can help to improve our sleep patterns by inducing a natural tiredness. However, it is wise not to exercise too close to bedtime as this can cause sleep disturbances.
- **Distraction:** Exercise offers a distraction to our daily worries and stops us focusing on our mood.
- **Time out:** Exercise and physical activity offer 'time out' for us. They provide a distraction from our mood and the preoccupations and worries of our lives, and offer space for more positive thinking patterns to grow.

- **Weight management:** Physical activity and exercise help us to burn off some of the calories from the food that we eat. Medication to treat depression can sometimes contribute to unexplained weight gain – it has not been determined whether this is because it causes you to eat more, feel too tired and lethargic to exercise, or for some other reason. The main thing is that physical activity and exercise are effective weight-management tools.
- **Overall health and medical wellbeing:** Being physically active and exercising can help to prevent (and at the very least manage) some of the other diseases that may affect us (obesity, diabetes, coronary heart disease, high blood pressure, etc).
- **Social:** Exercise can be a great way to meet people.

Exercise and the mind

It is known that exercise and physical activity stimulate some of the chemicals in the brain that help to improve our mood and make us feel better.

Being physically active also reduces the harmful changes in both the brain and body caused by stress and depression. Physical activity and exercise offer an outlet to release tension: as we move, our joints become less stiff and our muscles use up the energy we have accumulated. Plus, when we are moving, our mind has a different focus.

> How to get started

This part of the book contains different exercise plans that you can do at home, or outdoors if you prefer, along with some suggestions for other types of exercise. The exercises can be done for 5 or 30 minutes, so you can adapt them to suit you. These are ideal for exercising in private, but don't forget that there are other options.

If you want to get out and about, classes at leisure centres, gyms or studios cater for all tastes, ages and levels of fitness. You don't have to do kick-boxing or intense aerobics: there are Pilates or yoga classes where students are encouraged to go at their own pace, or you could try aqua aerobics – a fun and gentle form of exercise. Or why not join a dancing class? The added bonus is that you can take a breather when you need to.

Don't be put off by the idea that everyone at the gym or in a class is really fit either. Most classes will be full of red-faced, out-of-breath people having a good time. The ideal attitude is to give it your best shot and forget about appearances.

If you're in any doubt that the class is right for you, try to get in touch with the instructor and have a talk with them beforehand. They will let you know what level of fitness is required, and help you make a choice that suits you.

> I have worked with loads of people in the gym who thought that the place was going to be full of intimidatingly fit people – they are always so relieved to discover that gyms are full of real people like them and me!

Debbie, aged 45, fitness instructor

Safety first

Before going any further, you need to run through a few questions designed to highlight any health problems that might affect your ability to exercise.

Take a look at the table opposite, and tick 'yes' or 'no' as appropriate.

There are plenty of options for people with health conditions or a low level of fitness, so don't be down-hearted if you answered 'yes' to any of these questions. From exercise classes designed specifically for older people to gentle chair-based exercises (see page 69) to swimming, there will be something for you. The main thing is that you approach any new exercise with an understanding of your physical condition and limitations – that way you can exercise at a level that's safe and rewarding for you.

Are you fit to get physical?		yes	no
1	Has your doctor ever said you have a heart or vascular condition and/or that you should only do activity recommended or supervised by a doctor?		
2	Do you feel any pain in your chest when you do physical activity?		
3	In the past month have you had chest pain when you were not doing physical activity?		
4	Do you lose your balance because of dizziness or ever lose consciousness?		
5	Do you have a bone or joint problem that could be made worse by physical activity?		
6	Is your doctor currently prescribing medication for any condition?		
7	Are you over 69 years of age and not used to physical activity?		
8	Do you know of any reason why you should not take part in physical activity?		
9	Are you pregnant now or have you been pregnant in the last six months?		
10	Have you been diagnosed with a medical condition in the last two months?		
11	Are you significantly overweight?		

If you have answered yes to any of these questions please discuss the answers with your doctor who will advise you on whether it is the right time to become more active.

If you answered no to all of them, you are ready to up your exercise and activity levels.

> Know your medication: some medicines can have an effect on your heart rate, blood pressure and energy levels as well as contributing to weight gain. If in doubt, discuss your medication with your GP.

My mum is 65 years old. She walks her dog every day, shops and cleans for her older brothers and sisters and manages my garden as well as her own. I am always amazed at how this woman climbs ladders, washes windows and chops down trees!

My dad, who is now 78, became very inactive shortly after retiring. He sat watching TV and having tea made for him – he just did not move much. Then, at age of 72, one of life's bombshells hit him: his marriage broke down and he had to move into sheltered housing. He went to the GP because he was feeling depressed and his doctor prescribed some medication. More importantly, though, he advised my father to start exercising.

Dad joined the local gym, which offered a special membership fee for senior members. He now goes to the gym every day and has a circle of friends (all the young Mums – they get on like a house on fire!) He tells me, 'I don't push myself. I have 30 minutes on the rower, then 30 minutes on the treadmill, then I do some weights.' I dread to think what he would be doing if he did push himself! Last year he proudly showed me the gym newsletter: he was 'member of the month'.

Dad still gets the blues sometimes – when he thinks that life 'has not turned out the way it should have' – but he knows that going to the gym has made a big difference for him. I've taken a leaf out of his book too.

Jonathon, aged 45

> How often should I exercise?

The idea is that you can build an increase in physical activity into your life very easily, whether you're walking to work or doing some simple exercises. But how much should you do?

Targets to work towards	
Frequency	Aim to be active on at least 5 days of the week. You can start with 1 day a week at first and build up.
Intensity	When you are moving, you need to work at a level where you feel a little breathless but comfortable. This will be different for each person: some people may find walking up the stairs easy and some may find it hard work.
Time	Being active for 30 minutes each day is ideal. You can break this down into shorter intervals throughout the day: try a short 10-minute walk, and repeat it 3 times during the day.
Type	Choose any activity that fits well into your daily lifestyle, that you like doing and that you know you have the potential to keep up. Remember that this can be walking the dog, gardening or cleaning the house too!

> How hard should I work?

When you are taking part in physical activity and exercise, it is essential to monitor how hard you are working. The scale shown in the table on page 64 provides a useful way for you to check that you are working at the right level. It can help you to recognise how much energy you are putting in to the activity/exercise.

Working at the right level		
Number rating	How it feels for you?	
1	Very light	I could keep this going all day
2	Light	I feel a little warmer
3	Moderate	I can feel my heart beating a bit faster and I am breathing heavier
4	Somewhat hard	This feels harder but I am still comfortable
5	Getting harder	I am really feeling it now but not too bad
6	Hard	Ooh, this is barely comfortable
7	Harder	Uncomfortable now, I can't do this for long
8	Very hard	Very uncomfortable and I cannot keep going
9	Very, very hard	I need to stop, this feels awful
10	Maximum	I'm about to collapse

Aim to work at a level between 3 and 4 when performing activities
Aim to work at a level between 3 and 5 when exercising

Be patient with your levels of motivation. Even a little is better than nothing! Simply taking one small step towards being more active will make a difference to how you feel, providing a shift from your current physical state. Be sensitive to your energy levels too. You can build up your activity levels by doing 5 minutes at a time and then resting. Build up to 30 minutes at your own pace and in your own time.

>> Posture

When exercising, it's important to start from a position of good posture. However, posture is important at all times. Bad posture can affect the functioning of our inner organs, and sitting in a slumped position will promote shallow and ineffective breathing patterns, which may contribute to a lack of confidence and maintain our low mood. And poor posture can also lead to permanent problems in later life and contribute to back pain.

Standing and moving with correct posture can also lead to greater confidence. Open posture is expansive; hunched-over posture gives the appearance of closing in on oneself.

STANDING POSTURE

You can do this in front of a mirror or maybe ask a friend to check how you are standing. Standing side-on, you should be able to visualise a straight line running from your ear lobe to the middle of your ankle. Your body should be upright, without leaning back or forwards and without any excessive rounding or hollowing of the spine.

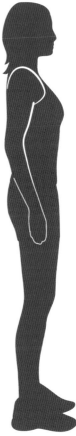

- Stand with your feet parallel and hip-width apart
- Distribute your weight between heel bone, big toe and little toe
- Spread your toes, aligning second toe with knee and hip
- Find a neutral pelvic position – it should not be tipped forwards or backwards
- Lengthen your torso and neck
- Tighten your deeper abdominal (tummy) muscles by visualising that you are zipping up a tight pair of trousers
- Look forwards, keeping your chin parallel to the floor
- Keeping your shoulders relaxed, slide your shoulder blades down towards your buttocks
- Keep your hands by the sides of your body, palms facing forwards.

SEATED POSTURE

It is important to sit correctly, particularly when we are working at a desk, to prevent low back pain – sitting correctly also enables us to breathe more fully.

- Sit towards the front of your chair
- Place your feet parallel and hip-width apart with knees over ankles
- Distribute your weight evenly between heel bone, big toe and little toe
- Spread your toes
- Lift up out of your sitting bones to find a neutral pelvic position
- Lengthen your torso and neck
- Tighten your abdominals by pulling in your tummy
- Look forwards, keeping your chin parallel to the floor
- Slide your shoulder blades down keeping them relaxed
- Place your hands by the sides of the chair.

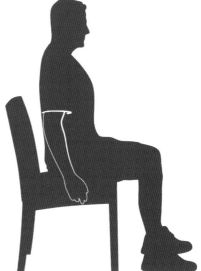

Finding a neutral pelvic position

Tilt or rock your pelvis gently forwards to hollow your back and then gently backwards to flatten your back. Find the middle between these two extremes – this is your *neutral pelvic position*.

Instant relief

Stop what you are doing right now and open your posture. Notice how much better it feels to lengthen your spine, lift your head and slide your shoulder blades down. Like smiling when you feel low, changing your posture can really improve your mood.

Exercise programmes

It's time to get started. There are lots of different kinds of exercises illustrated in this section. From chair-based exercises suitable for the workplace (see page 69) to the high-energy cardiovascular workout on page 83, you should be able to pick and mix a routine that suits your mood.

If you are not used to exercise, select *one* of the routines to start with – ideally the warm-up routine – and practise a couple of exercises at first. Then gradually add in more when you feel ready for a longer workout. You can mix and match exercises from the different routines to design your own workout. Keep your legs moving all the time using marching or walking on the spot if you can, and substitute this for any exercises you find too challenging.

It's important that you work at a pace and level that suit you. Listen to your body and adjust your workout accordingly. It's far better to start with a few easy exercises that you find comfortable and do them well and often, than try to do everything at once and give up in exhaustion.

Always remember to warm up first, and it's a good idea to cool down with stretches at the end. You should aim to begin gently, work a little harder in the middle and then gradually work down.

Note: All routines can vary in length, depending on how many repetitions of each exercise you do, and how many exercises you choose to perform. A good starting point is 5 to 10 minutes of the mobility and warming routine – then add in other exercises as you see fit.

Safety Tips

Before you start exercising, you need to make sure you follow some safety guidance first:

- First complete the questionnaire (on page 61) to check you're fit to get exercising.
- When you are exercising wear loose-fitting, comfortable clothing and a supportive, comfortable pair of trainers.
- If you are exercising outdoors, make sure you wear appropriate clothing and take precautions to keep warm or protect yourself against the environment (use sunscreen in summer). For personal safety, always take a mobile phone with you and make sure you tell someone where you are going and what time you will return.
- If you feel thirsty, sip water throughout, but avoid taking long drinks.
- If you have eaten a heavy meal, wait two hours before exercising.
- If you want to exercise but feel hungry, have a light snack like a banana or a piece of toast. It is useful to have a small snack immediately after any activity to provide the nutrients you need to replenish your energy stores.
- Only do what feels comfortable. If anything feels uncomfortable, don't do it. It just means that it may not be right for your body.
- Remember that the suggested time and number of repetitions in the exercises that follow are a guide only, and should be adapted to suit yor level of fitness.
- Only exercise when you feel well and healthy. Do not exercise if you have a cold or flu or if you are excessively tired.
- Make sure there is enough space around you. Move any chairs, tables or bags out of the way.
- Check your posture before you start (see page 65).
- Breathe naturally at all times and never hold your breath.
- Always complete the warm-up before you move on to the cardiovascular, strengthening or stretching exercises.
- Try to complete the stretching focus at the end of your routine.

DESK RELIEF EXERCISES

Many of us spend a great deal of time sitting at a desk or in a chair. This can contribute to stiffness and tension. This section describes a simple routine of six exercises that can be practised anytime, anywhere, to help you feel more relaxed and flexible. You can even do these in bed, or while watching TV.

For all seated exercises start from a position of good posture. You should have a straight back with your tummy tucked in, your neck long, shoulders relaxed and your feet hip-width apart.

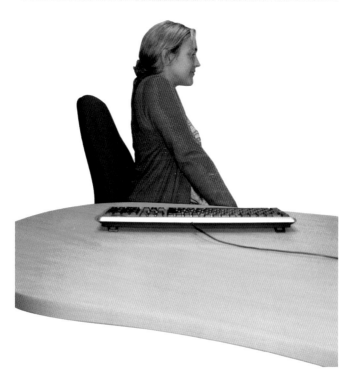

Shoulder rolls

1. SHOULDER ROLLS

❶ Maintain an upright posture and engage your abdominals
❷ Roll your shoulders forwards, upwards, backwards and down
❸ Perform 8–12 repetitions

2. SIDE BENDS

❶ Lift your torso and bend to one side in a controlled manner
❷ Return to the central position
❸ Lift and bend to the other side in a controlled manner
❹ Return to the central position
❺ Only bend as far over as is comfortable
❻ Visualise your body as being placed between two panes of glass
   as you bend
❼ Perform 8–12 repetitions

3. SIDE TWISTS

❶ Hold your arms comfortably in front of you at shoulder level, with
   the elbows slightly bent
❷ Twist around to one side
❸ Come gently back to the centre
❹ Then twist to the other side
❺ Keep your hips facing forwards
❻ Keep your chest lifted and shoulders relaxed and down
❼ Perform 8–12 repetitions

4. CHAIR MARCHING

❶ Sit upright with your feet hip-width apart, knees bent and
   abdominals engaged
❷ March your legs gently, maintaining an upright posture
❸ Keep this going for one minute, have a rest then repeat

5. HEEL DIGS

1 Dig alternate heels to the floor in front of your body, maintaining an upright posture

2 Keep this going for one minute, have a rest then repeat

6. CHEST STRETCH

1 Take your hands behind you and hold the back of your chair or seat

2 Lean forwards slightly until a mild tension is felt at the front of the chest

3 Keep your elbows slightly bent

4 Squeeze your shoulder blades together and lift your chest to increase the stretch

5 Hold the stretch for 8–12 seconds

Note: Your hands can also be placed on your buttocks or clasped together behind your back – whichever is most comfortable.

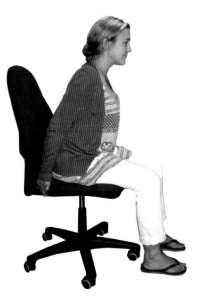

Chest stretch

WARM UP

These standing exercises are designed to loosen the joints and give a better range of movement. They prevent the body becoming stiff and immobile and also help to improve posture. Some of the movements will get the muscles warm and increase the heart rate and may activate the release of endorphins – the feel-good hormones. Remember to start from a good posture position with your back straight and your tummy tucked in, and breathe naturally throughout.

1. SHOULDER ROLLS

1 Gently roll your shoulders forwards, then up and backwards and finally downwards

2 As you lower your shoulders, feel your shoulder blades slide down towards your buttocks

3 Perform 8–12 repetitions

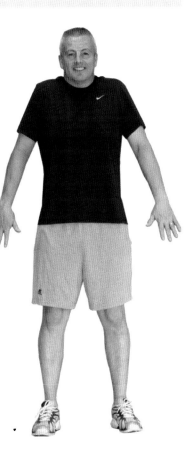

2. SIDE BENDS

1. Bend directly to the side in a controlled manner and return to the central position
2. Bend directly to the other side in a controlled manner and return to the central position
3. Visualise your body as being placed between two panes of glass and bend only as far over as is comfortable
4. Keep your hips facing forwards and the movement controlled
5. Keep your body lifted between the hips and the ribs
6. Perform 8–16 repetitions on each side (alternating)

3. SIDE TWISTS

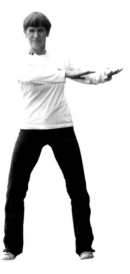

1. Start with your feet shoulder-width apart
2. Hold out your arms at shoulder level, with your elbows slightly bent or place your hands on hips
3. Twist around to one side, back to the centre and then twist to the other side
4. Twist only as far around as is comfortable
5. Keep your hips and knees facing forwards
6. Perform 8–16 repetitions on each side (alternating)

4. LEG CURLS

❶ Start with your feet shoulder-width apart
❷ Step out to the right and transfer your weight over to your right leg, kicking your left heel towards the buttocks
❸ Step your left leg down and transfer your weight onto this leg, kicking your right heel to the buttocks
❹ Take a large but comfortable stride of the legs
❺ Keep your hips facing forwards and avoid hollowing the lower back by tightening your abdominal muscles
❻ Ensure that your knee joint remains unlocked when landing
❼ Keep the movement controlled, smooth and not jerky
❽ Perform 8–16 repetitions on each side (alternating)

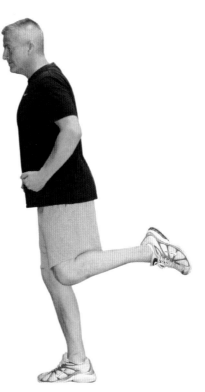

5. HEEL AND TOE

1. Start with your feet shoulder-width apart and take your weight onto one leg
2. Dig the heel of your free foot towards the floor and then point the toe towards the floor
3. Keep your weight-bearing leg soft, your hips facing forwards and the movement controlled
4. Aim for the heel and toe to land in the same place
5. Repeat on the other leg
6. Perform 8–16 repetitions on each side (alternating)

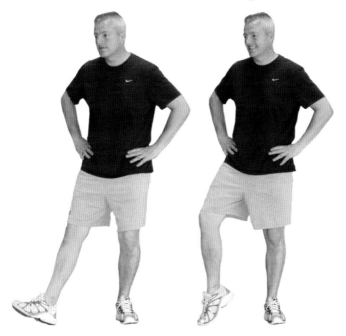

6. KNEE LIFTS

1 Start with your feet shoulder-width apart
2 Start raising alternate knees in front of your body
3 Take a comfortable stride of the legs
4 Keep your hips facing forwards
5 Lift your leg only to a height that is comfortable and keep your back straight
6 Keep your chest lifted and do not allow your body to bend forwards as your leg lifts
7 Perform for 1–2 minutes

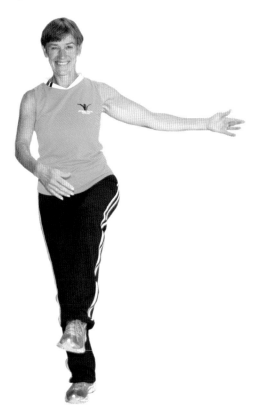

7. MARCHING/WALKING

1 Start with your feet hip-width apart

2 Maintain an upright posture and engage your abdominals

3 Start marching or walking on the spot

4 Land your feet lightly

5 Keep your knees unlocked

6 You can play music and march for as long as you like

7 You can also travel this movement forwards and backwards or around the room

8 Perform for 2–4 minutes

Note: Marching can be used as a warm-up in its own right. It will raise your heart rate and warm your muscles. It can also be used between exercises, or in breaks between repetitions of exercises as you build up stamina.

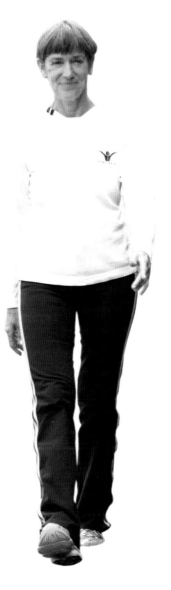

STRETCH IT OUT

These exercises reduce any tightness and can lengthen the muscles. Lengthening the muscles helps to reduce tension (a postural shift than can improve mood). This improve the efficiency of our movements and can make daily tasks easier. Stretching also assists with relaxation and can improve posture. It's a good idea to stretch after a warm-up and before moving on to other exercises. Stretching is also an important part of the warm-down. Only stretch as far as is comfortable and remember to hold a stretch – don't bounce.

1. HAMSTRINGS STRETCH

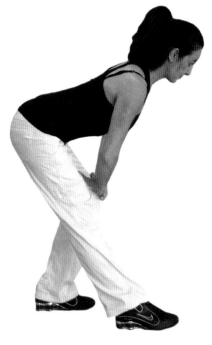

1 Step one leg forwards

2 Bend the knee of your back leg and place your hands at the top of your thigh of the bent knee

3 Bend forwards from the hips, supporting your weight with your hands

4 Stop when a mild tension is felt at the back of the thigh of the straight leg

5 Keep the knee of your straight leg fully extended, but not locked out

6 Keep your spine long and your chest lifted

7 Hold the stretch for 10–15 seconds

8 Repeat on the other leg

2. QUADRICEPS STRETCH

1 Balance on one leg – use a wall or chair to support you
2 Raise the opposite foot towards your buttocks until a mild tension
is felt at the front of the thigh
3 Use your hand to hold the leg in
place
4 Keep your supporting knee joint
unlocked
5 Make sure your heel lifts
towards the centre of your body,
not to the side
6 Tilt your pelvis slightly forwards
7 Keep both knee joints in line
with each other
8 Hold the stretch for 10–15
seconds
9 Repeat on the other leg

3. CALF STRETCH

1 Step your right leg backwards as far as possible and with the heel
of this back foot on the floor
2 Keep your front knee bent but do not let your knee roll inwards
3 Keep your hips
facing forwards
4 Visualise a straight
line running from
your ear to the ankle
of your extended leg
5 Use a wall or chair
to support you
6 Hold the stretch for
10–15 seconds
7 Repeat on the
other leg

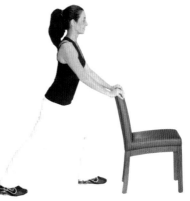

4. ADDUCTOR STRETCH

1. Lunge to the side, taking your body weight onto the bent leg
2. Keep your other leg extended, knee straight but not locked
3. Keep the hips facing forwards and avoid hollowing the lower back
4. Use a wall for support if you need to
5. Hold the stretch for 10–15 seconds
6. Repeat on the other leg

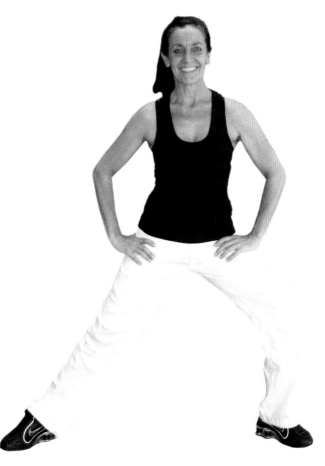

5. OBLIQUES STRETCH

① Start with your feet shoulder width and a half apart

② Place one hand on your hip to support your body weight

③ Raise your other arm up and bend over slightly to the side

④ Keep the knee joint of both legs slightly bent

⑤ Emphasise lifting your body upwards rather than leaning too far over to the side

⑥ Stretch only to a point where a mild tension is felt at the side of your trunk

⑦ Keep your body weight equally placed between your legs and avoid pushing your hip out to the side

⑧ When bending to the side, move your body in a straight line and without leaning forwards or backwards

⑨ Hold the stretch for 10–15 seconds

⑩ Repeat on the other side

6. TRICEPS STRETCH

1. Start with your feet shoulder-width apart
2. Place one hand over your head on the centre of your back
3. Use your other arm to ease the arm further down
4. Hold the position with your knees slightly bent
5. Stretch to a point where a mild tension is felt at the back of your upper arm
6. Hold the stretch for 10–15 seconds
7. Repeat on the other arm

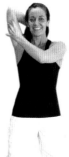

7. CHEST STRETCH

1. Start with your feet shoulder-width apart
2. Take your hands backwards until a mild tension is felt at the front of your chest – your hands can be placed on your buttocks or clasped together behind your back, whichever is most comfortable
3. Keep your knees unlocked
4. Keep your elbows slightly bent
5. Slide your shoulder blades down and lift your chest to increase the stretch
6. Hold the stretch for 10–15 seconds

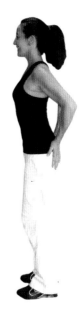

CARDIO

This cardiovascular routine is designed to make the heart and circulatory system stronger. It will also contribute to the release of endorphins providing the feel-good factor, which can last for a long time after the initial activity has ended. It's important to perform five minutes of warm-up exercises first and ideally some stretches too. Start gently, work harder in the middle then ease up. Take care doing impact exercises like jogging if you have joint problems, and always go at your own speed.

1. MARCH OR JOG ON THE SPOT

Jogging and marching on the spot can help keep you warm between exercises. They are also great cardiovascular activities in their own right too. Depending on your level of fitness, use marching or jogging for a few minutes on their own; to keep you warm between exercises; or as a break between repetitions of the same exercise.

2. SQUATS WITH ARM CIRCLES

1. Start with your feet two hip-widths apart, so that when you bend your knees they stay in line with your toes
2. Bend your knees to a 90-degree angle
3. Straight then again without locking your knees
4. Add a circling movement of your arms in front of your body to raise the intensity
5. Start with 30 seconds and then march for 30 seconds

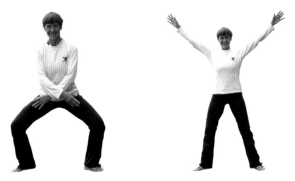

3. LUNGES

❶ Maintain an upright
posture and engage your
abdominals
❷ Lunge to the side, keeping
your hips facing forwards
❸ Step back and repeat
❹ Start with 30 seconds and
then go back to marching
or jogging for 30 seconds

Note: you can add some
forward or backward lunges
to vary your routine

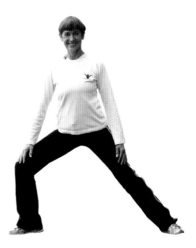

4. LEG KICKS

❶ Kick alternate legs out in front
of your body
❷ You can add a hop at the
same time if it feels
comfortable
❸ Keep your hopping knee joint
unlocked and make sure your
heel goes down
❹ Take care not to lock the knee
of your kicking leg
❺ Start with 30 seconds, then
march for 30 seconds to
reduce the impact on the joints

Note: Gradually build up the
number of cycles of kicking and
marching and increase the
number of seconds for each.

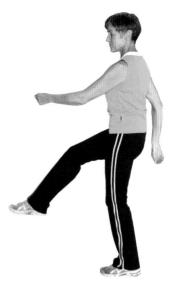

5. TRAVELLING SIDE SQUATS

1 Start with your feet shoulder-width apart
2 Step one leg to the side in a squat and then travel the other leg in the same direction to stand upright
3 Repeat 4 times moving to the right and 4 times moving back to the left
4 Keep your hips facing forwards
5 Take care not to squat too deeply – maintain a 90-degree angle at the knees
6 Perform for 1–2 minutes

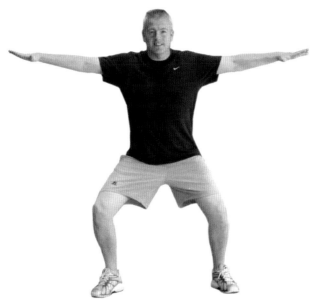

Cardio exercises can help tone the muscles of the lower body, release muscle tension and maintain a healthy body weight. If you don't want to perform these exercises then walking is also a great cardiovascular activity, with the added advantage of getting you outdoors in the fresh air.

GET STRONG

You can perform these strengthening exercises after you have finished the cardiovascular exercises or the warm-up, if you feel like a longer workout. When you have finished, stretch all the muscles while you are nice and warm. Correct breathing is very important: the main thing is not to hold your breath. Ideally, you should breathe out on the effort – the lifting phase of the movement – and breathe in on the lowering phase of the exercise.

1. DEAD-LIFT WITH WEIGHTS

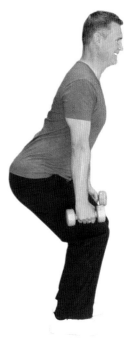

1 Stand upright with your feet hip-width apart

2 Bend at the knees and hips – but don't curve your back – as though you are reaching to lift something from the floor

3 Return to an upright position by straightening your knees and hips and leading with your shoulders

4 Push your buttocks backwards and don't let your knees travel too far forwards

5 Your bottom should be higher than your knees when bending

6 Look forwards and slightly upwards

7 If the exercise feels easy, try lifting a small weight from the floor

8 Start with 8 repetitions and gradually build up to 16–24

Note: You should use this action when lifting any object from the floor.

2. UPRIGHT ROW WITH WEIGHTS

1 Maintain an upright posture with your knees slightly bent, feet hip-width apart

2 Lift up the dumbbells to chest level, keeping them close to your body

3 Lower them down under control

4 Start with 8 repetitions and gradually build up to 16–24

Note: if you don't have dumbbells you can use cans of baked beans or water bottles.

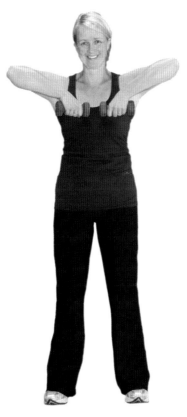

3. SIT-UPS/CURL-UPS

1. Lie on your back with your knees bent and your feet firmly on the floor
2. Place your hands on your thighs or at the sides of your head
3. Engage your abdominal muscles by pulling in your tummy
4. Use your tummy muscles to curl your shoulders and chest off the floor
5. Lift as far as is comfortable, but without lifting your lower back off the floor
6. Lower yourself down under control
7. Keep your neck relaxed throughout and look forwards
8. Start with 8 repetitions and gradually build up to 16–20

Note: placing your hands across your chest or at the sides of your head makes this exercise harder – don't pull at your head as you lift up.

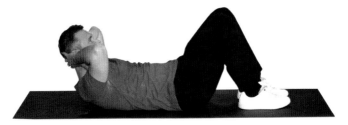

These strengthening activities can help tone and shape the muscles. They also provide a release from any tension and improve the posture. Remember to breathe naturally throughout, using the out breath to help you.

4. BACK EXTENSIONS

1. Lie face down on the floor and rest your hands at your side on the floor
2. Engage your abdominals lightly and contract your back muscles
3. Raise your chest away from the floor, keeping your neck in line with the rest of your spine
4. Lower back down to the floor slowly
5. Start with 8 repetitions and gradually build up to 16–20

Note: you can also put your hands on your buttocks or at the sides of your head to make this harder.

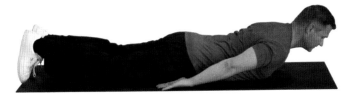

> After I had my fourth child I suffered from post-natal depression for a few months. Even though my friends, family and GP were very supportive, I couldn't shake off the feelings of helplessness and anger. Then my sister came to stay. She won't take 'no' for an answer, and frog-marched me to the gym, to dance classes and even horse-riding. At first I was outraged, but then I remembered that before I had my children I really enjoyed being active. For me, this was the key to my recovery: it gave me an outlet for my emotions, helped me deal with my body-image issues, and allowed me some time for myself. Although I adore my children, I wouldn't give up my precious exercise time for any of them!

Lynn, aged 40

5. PRESS-UPS

1 Take up a full plank position with your body straight, supported on your arms and toes
2 Your hands should be a shoulder width and a half apart
3 Make sure that your shoulders are forward of the hands
4 Engage your abdominals
5 Bend your elbows to lower your chest towards the wall or floor
6 Extend your elbows to return to the start position
7 Keep your elbows unlocked
8 Start with 8 repetitions and gradually build up to 16–20

Note: you can rest whenever you need to – press-ups are hard! If you prefer, you can do a slightly easier version with your knees bent and resting on the floor, or you can take up a standing position and do press-ups against a wall.

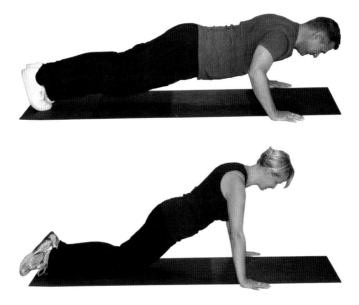

6. CALF RAISE

1 Stand with your feet hip-width apart and engage your abdominals
2 Rest your hands lightly on a chair back if you need support
3 Rise onto the balls of your feet, lifting your heels from the floor
4 Lower your heels under control
5 Keep your knee joints unlocked
6 Start with 8–12 repetitions and gradually build up to 16–24

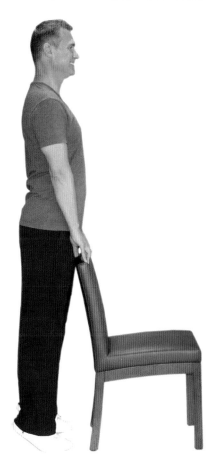

7. BICEPS CURL WITH WEIGHTS

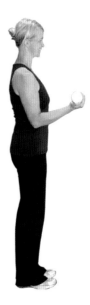

❶ Stand with your feet hip-width apart and
engage your abdominals
❷ Fix your elbows in to the sides of your body
❸ Raise the dumbbells in an arc-like motion
towards your chest
❹ Lower them under control without locking
your elbows
❺ Keep your wrists fixed and straight
❻ Your lower arms should be the only body
parts moving
❼ Start with 8–12 repetitions and gradually
build up to 16–24

Note: if you do not have dumbbells, use a can
of baked beans.

8. OUTER-THIGH RAISES

❶ Lie on one side, engage your abdominals and bend the bottom
knee to assist balance
❷ Raise and lower your top leg slowly
❸ Keep your hips facing forwards as you lift your leg up
❹ When the exercise feels easy, you can rest and then perform
another set
❺ Start with 8–12 repetitions and gradually build up to 16–24

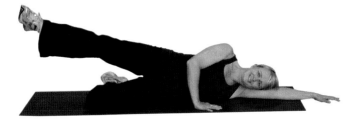

9. INNER-THIGH RAISES

1. Lie on one side and bend your top knee across your body to rest it on the floor
2. Raise and lower your bottom leg slowly
3. Lift your leg without moving your waist or rolling your hips backwards
4. Start with 8–12 repetitions and gradually build up to 16–24

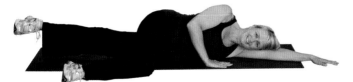

Thank you for reading

We hope you feel inspired by this book to exercise a little more, and have realised how simple it can be. Whether you give yourself ten minutes of chair-based exercises at work, or feel inspired to put on some music and work your way through a half-hour energetic cardio routine, you will start to feel the benefits almost at once.

But exercise at home isn't for everyone. Some people prefer to get out of the house into the fresh air, or out with some company. You can do some of these exercises as you walk or jog around the park – just make sure you feel nicely warm beforehand.

Or maybe you prefer a completely different option? Turn over for some of our favourite suggestions. Now go and enjoy yourself!

Swimming

Water is a naturally relaxing environment and swimming is a great form of exercise. It promotes the circulation of blood and gets rid of any unused energy and mental tension. The pressure of water provides a massaging effect, and its buoyancy automatically reduces some of the physical stress on the body. This makes it a good option if you have joint problems or a low level of fitness, and want to steer clear of high-impact exercises.

There is also some evidence that immersion in water will calm the part of the nervous system that speeds up during times of stress. This means there are real benefits for your state of mind, even as you tone your body and improve your cardiovascular fitness.

If you aren't a good swimmer then consider taking classes at your local pool – it's never too late to start. Or you could opt for an aqua aerobics class. These are a fun way to exercise, with a trained instructor and a relaxing, non-competitive environment.

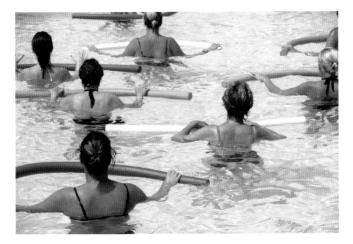

> Dancing

Dance is a cardiovascular activity with many health benefits. There are so many types of dance that there's really something for everyone: from Ballroom to Tango, Salsa to Jive, a dance class is a wonderful way to get yourself moving and have fun in the process. It's also a very sociable activity and a great way to break down barriers.

If you're not quite ready to dance in public, then all you have to do is clear some space, put on some music and move. There are no rules – anything goes! Whether you've just come home from work, are getting ready to go out or are dancing round the house while doing the dusting, it'll give your mood an instant lift.

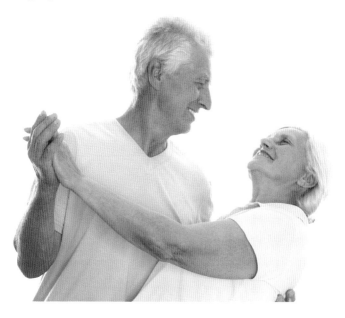

>> # Yoga

Yoga is a form of exercise that increases flexibility and promotes strength and balance. Some classes can be quite strenuous while others focus on gentle movements and breathing techniques. If you're interested in taking a class there are usually plenty of options, but try to speak to the instructor and find out if this is the right one for you.

Many people find that yoga not only gives them a greater level of strength and suppleness, but that is also helps them relax and focus. This makes it incredibly beneficial if you have a stressful lifestyle. Another advantage is that yoga can be practised in your own home – all you need is a mat and some loose-fitting clothing. People who start learning yoga as beginners soon feel ready to practise on their own. It is a great tool for taking control and learning to relax.

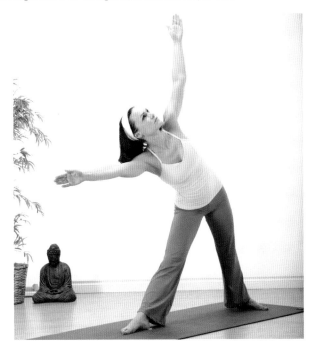

Walking

> If I could not walk far and fast, I think I should just explode and perish.
>
> **Charles Dickens**

Walking offers a great way to improve cardiovascular fitness. It's easy and accessible, and there are many different ways to do it: you can walk round a park, walk briskly through the streets or head for the countryside. Walking can be enjoyed alone or with friends, and can be combined with other pleasures such as visiting a National Trust property or walking to a country pub for lunch.

If you want company on your walk there are plenty of groups you can join: there are organised sight-seeing walks in most cities; you can contact a group like the Ramblers; or you can look out for nature walks in your local area.

If you are new to walking you might want to start with a short walk once a week and progressively build up the time you spend walking. Even a 15-minute walk to the shops can improve your fitness, and it's therapeutic too. Most problems can be put in perspective during a walk.

> The moment my legs begin to move, my thoughts begin to flow.
>
> **Henry David Thoreau**

When I retired, my children went on at me about getting exercise and taking care of myself. They suggested all sorts of things like joining a gym or going to yoga or Pilates – even ballroom dancing was mentioned. But I didn't really feel like making a fool of myself at 66, so I ignored them.

They were right though: before long, I found it difficult to get through the days. I felt busy but useless, stressed yet lacking in purpose. Then a neighbour of mine suggested that I accompany her on a walk one day. She's part of a group called the Saturday Walkers Club that meets every week in a different place to walk, talk and have a pub lunch. I discovered that though I didn't want to take an exercise class or join a gym, I loved these walks through the country. I always returned from them as relaxed and focused as I had felt tired and stressed beforehand. I honestly believe now that there's no problem – big or small – that doesn't get fixed when you take a long walk in good company.

Alex, aged 67

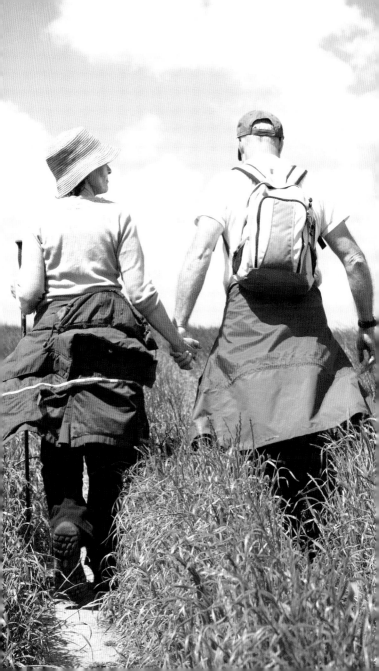

appendices

> > ## Appendix 1: Activity Log

This can help you to monitor and build your activity levels.

- Start by writing down your current activity levels
- Write down one small change you would like to make to your activity levels on one day
- Make that change and monitor your progress
- When you feel ready, progressively add in more changes on more days

Day / Date	6am–8am	8am–10am	10am–12	12–2pm	2pm–4pm	4pm–6pm	6pm–8pm	8pm–10pm
Example	Walk to station	Desk exercises		Go for a walk in lunch hour		Walk home from station	Pilates class or swimming	
Monday								
Tuesday								
Wednesday								
Thursday								
Friday								
Saturday								
Sunday								

>> Appendix 2: Food and mood diary

You can use a food diary to monitor and make changes to your eating patterns. You can also use the diary to make a note of how your mood affects your eating. This can then help you to look at other strategies you can use to improve your mood and manage your eating.

- Start by writing down everything you eat and drink for one or two days
- Write down one small change you would like to make to your eating habits on one day
- Make that change and monitor your progress
- When you feel ready, progressively build in more changes on more days

Day/Date	Breakfast	Mid-morning snack	Lunch	Mid-afternoon snack	Dinner	Evening snack
Food	Skipped breakfast Cup of coffee	2 cups of coffee and biscuits	Sardines on toast and coffee	Chocolate bar and 2 cups of coffee	2 glasses of wine Spaghetti Bolognese	
Mood	Stressed – woke up late	Tired	OK	Angry at boss for giving me another job to finish. Knew I would finish work late again!	Relieved to be home	Tired
Change I would like to make		Take some fruit to eat at break			Drink a glass of water and drink wine after dinner, not before	

Appendix 3: Sleep record

Use this to record your current sleeping patterns and identify any factors that may prevent you from sleeping. You can then find strategies to help to improve your sleep, such as taking a notebook to record worrying thoughts, eating earlier or not drinking a stimulant (e.g. coffee) before you go to bed.

- Start by making a note of your current sleeping patterns
- Identify any potential causes or contributory factors
- Decide if there are any actions you can take to start improving the quality of your sleep

Day	Monday	Tuesday	Wednesday	Thursday	Friday	Saturday	Sunday
Sleep			Interrupted		Heavy		Interrupted
Concerns or worries			Home late from work, ate late		Drank a lot of alcohol		Worrying about jobs to do
Strategy			Be assertive Leave work on time Take a lunch time walk				Have a notebook beside the bed to write down thoughts

bibliography

ACSM (2005) 7th edition. *ACSM's Guidelines for Exercise Testing and Prescription*. USA. Lippincott, Williams & Wilkins.

Benson, H, MD (1975). *The Relaxation Response*. New York. Avon books.

Biddle, S, Fox, K & Boutcher, S (2000) Eds. *Physical Activity and Psychological Well-Being*. London and New York. Routledge.

Bird, W (2007). 'Natural Thinking: A Report for the Royal Society for the Protection of Birds Investigating the Links Between the Natural Environment, Biodiversity and Mental Health'. Available from www.rspb.org.uk.

Borg G (1998). *Perceived Exertion and Pain Scales*. USA. Human Kinetics.

British Nutrition Foundation (2005). 'Balance of Good Health'. Available from: www.nutrition.org.uk.

Department of Health (2004). 'At Least Five a Week: Evidence on the Impact of Physical Activity and Its Relationship to Health. A report from the Chief Medical Officer'. London. Department of Health.

Department of Health (2004). 'Choosing Health: Making Healthier Choices Easier'. London. Department of Health.

Durstine, L J & Moore, G (2003) 2nd edition. *ACSM's Exercise Management for Persons with Chronic Diseases and Disabilities*. USA. Human Kinetics.

Feltham, C & Horton, I (2000) Eds. *Handbook of Counselling and Psychotherapy*. UK. Sage publications.

Halliwell, E (2005). 'Up and Running? Exercise Therapy and the Treatment of Mild or Moderate Depression in Primary Care'. UK. Available from: www.mentalhealth.org.uk.

Hawton K & Simkin S (2003). 'Helping people bereaved by suicide'. *BMJ* 327: 177–178.

Ironside, V *You'll Get Over It: The Rage of Bereavement*. UK. Penguin Books Ltd.

Jeffers, S (1997). *Feel the Fear and do it Anyway*. UK. Rider & Co.

Johnston D & Mayers C (2005). 'Spirituality: A review of how occupational therapists acknowledge, assess and meet spiritual needs'. *BJOT* 68 (9): 386.

Jonas, S & Phillips, E (2009). *ACSM's Exercise is Medicine. A Clinicians Guide to Exercise Prescription*. Philadelphia. Lippincott, Williams and Wilkins.

Lago, C & Thompson, J (2003). *Race, Culture and Counselling*. Berkshire. Open University Press.

Lawrence, D (2004) 2nd edition. *The Complete Guide to Exercise in Water*. London. A&C Black.

Lawrence, D (2004) 2nd edition. *The Complete Guide to Exercise to Music*. London. A&C Black.

Lawrence, D & Hope, R (2005) 2nd edition. *The Complete Guide to Circuit Training*. London. A&C Black.

Lawrence, D & Barnett, L (2006). *GP referral Schemes*. London. A&C Black.

Max, D T (2010). 'The Secrets of Sleep'. *National Geographic Magazine*, May 2010.

PRODIGY (2005). 'Depression'. UK. Available from: www.prodigy.nhs.uk (accessed 28 August 2005).

Rogers, C & Stevens, B (1967). *Person To Person: The Problem of Being Human*. USA. Real People Press.

Royal College of Psychiatrists (2009). *The Young Mind: An Essential Guide to Mental Health for Young Adults, Parents and Teachers*. London. Bantam Press.

Scott Peck, M (1978). *The Road Less Travelled*. London. Random House Publishers.

Spearing, M (2002). 'Bipolar Disorder'. USA. Available from: www.nimh.nih.gov.

Stewart, I & Joines, V (1987). *TA Today. A New Introduction to Transactional Analysis*. Nottingham. Lifespace publishing.

Stock, M (2000). 'Depression'. USA. Available from: www.nimh.nih.gov.

Williams, C (2007). *Overcoming Anxiety*. UK. Hodder Arnold.

Williams, C (2007). *Overcoming Depression*. UK. Hodder Arnold.

find out more

Alcoholics Anonymous
www.alcoholics-anonymous.org.uk
Helpline: 0845 769 7555

Association for Post-Natal Illness
http://apni.org
Helpline: 020 7386 0868

Aware
Helping to defeat depression
www.aware.ie
Helpline: 00 353 1 90 303 302

British Snoring and Sleep Apnoea Association
www.britishsnoring.co.uk

Building exercise into your life
www.nhs.uk/change4life

Citizens Advice Bureau
www.adviceguide.org.uk
Helpline: 020 7833 2181

Cognitive Behavioural Therapy
Free life skills course
www.livinglifetothefull.com

British Association for Counselling
Search for a therapist
www.bacp.co.uk

Cruse Bereavement Care
www.crusebereavementcare.org.uk

Depression Alliance
www.depressionalliance.org

Depression UK
www.depressionuk.org

Drink Aware
www.drinkaware.co.uk

Drugs help and information
www.talktofrank.com

Family Action
Help tackling family problems
www.family-action.org.uk

Mental Health Foundation
Including food and mood information
www.mentalhealth.org.uk

MDF The Bipolar Organisation
www.mdf.org.uk
Helpline: 08456 340 540

National Debtline
www.nationaldebtline.co.uk
Helpline: 0808 808 4000

Relate
www.relate.org.uk
Tel: 0845 456 1310

Royal College of Psychiatrists
www.rcpsych.ac.uk

Sainsbury Centre for Mental Health
www.scmh.org.uk

Samaritans
www.samaritans.org
Helpline: 0845 790 9090

SaneLine
www.sane.org.uk
Tel: 0845 767 8000

Sleep Council
www.sleepcouncil.org.uk

Stop smoking
http://smokefree.nhs.uk

Walking for Health
www.wfh.naturalengland.org.uk

Young Minds
www.youngminds.org.uk
Tel: 020 7336 8445